Third Edition

Pharmacy Practice
for technicians
Workbook

Don A. Ballington, MS

Midlands Technical College
Columbia, South Carolina

Robert J. Anderson, PharmD

Mercer University Southern School of Pharmacy
Atlanta, Georgia

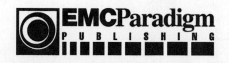

EMCParadigm
P U B L I S H I N G

Senior Editor	Christine Hurney
Developmental Editor	Cheryl Drivdahl
Editorial Assistant	Susan Capecchi
Copy Editor	Rich Cronin
Cover and Text Designer	Leslie Anderson
Desktop Production	Matthias Frasch
Proofreader	Judy Peacock

Publishing Management Team

Bob Cassel, Publisher; Jeanne Allison, Senior Acquisitions Editor; Janice Johnson, Vice President of Marketing; Shelley Clubb, Electronic Design and Production Manager

---

Text ISBN 0-7638-2226-4
Product Number 03659

Published by EMC Corporation
875 Montreal Way
St. Paul, MN 55102
(800) 535-6865
E-mail: educate@emcp.com
Web site: www.emcp.com

Printed in the United States of America.

10 9 8 7 6 5 4 3 2 1

UNIT 4 PROFESSIONALISM IN THE PHARMACY 175

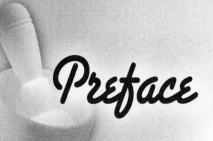

Preface

This workbook has been prepared to accompany the text *Pharmacy Practice for Technicians, Third Edition,* by Don A. Ballington and Robert J. Anderson. Along with the textbook, Encore CD, and supporting Internet Resource Center, this workbook is designed to help students learn techniques and procedures necessary to prepare and dispense medications in both community and institutional pharmacy settings.

This third edition of the workbook includes the following types of exercises:

- Communication and Pharmacy Practice questions offer students opportunities to review and apply chapter instruction. These questions help students understand the profession and business of pharmacy, laws and regulations that govern the profession, safe practices in community and hospital pharmacies, the types of information that can be communicated by pharmacy technicians and by pharmacists, and their own future in pharmacy practice.

- Mathematics Review exercises give students practice in using the pharmacy and business calculations presented in the textbook.

- Web Activities encourage research of resources and information available on the Internet.

- In the Lab activities for Units 2 and 3 allow students to apply what they have learned from the textbook in realistic community and hospital pharmacy situations. These activities include chances for interpreting medication orders, preparing medication labels, and keeping pharmacy records. They also offer practice in weighing and measuring pharmaceutical ingredients, compounding drugs, and preparing intravenous solutions.

- Puzzling Terminology crossword puzzles are fun features that reinforce chapter vocabulary and concepts as well as safe pharmacy practices.

Additional instructional support is provided on the Encore CD accompanying the textbook. Interactive Tech Check exercises allow students to review and apply chapter material by matching concepts from one column with corresponding concepts in another column. Interactive Review and Practice Test questions help students test their knowledge of concepts covered in the book. The questions are presented at two levels—book and chapter. Each level functions in two different modes: in the Review mode, students receive immediate feedback on each item and a report of their total score; in the Practice Test mode, the results are e-mailed to both students and their instructors.

The Encore CD includes a complete glossary with an image bank created from key illustrations in the textbook. To reinforce recognition of drug names, the Encore CD presents interactive flash cards of the top prescribed drugs.

The Internet Resource Center for this title at www.emcp.com provides additional chapter study resources, including PowerPoint slide shows as well as lecture and study notes. These resources can be downloaded and adapted to meet each student's particular study needs. The Internet Resource Center also offers crossword puzzles that provide practice on distinguishing brand names and generic names of the top prescribed drugs, and makes the interactive drug flash cards from the Encore CD available from any computer with an Internet connection.

The authors and editorial staff would like to thank Jennifer Danielson for creating instructional materials for Chapter 12, *Medication Safety*, and updating Chapter 14, *Your Future in Pharmacy Practice,* in this workbook. They would also like to thank Dr. Andrea Redman for her technical review.

The authors and editorial staff invite your feedback on the text and its supplements. Please reach us by clicking the "Contact Us" button at www.emcp.com.

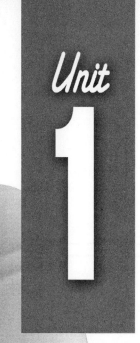

Unit 1

Principles of Pharmacy Practice

The Profession of Pharmacy

Chapter 1

COMMUNICATION AND PHARMACY PRACTICE

1. Define the following terms:

   a. paraprofessional _____
   _____

   b. accountability _____
   _____

   c. chronic _____
   _____

   d. unit dose _____
   _____

   e. galenical pharmacy ~~dose~~ the process of
   creating extracts of active medicinals from
   plants

2. Explain who these people were:

   a. Dioscorides wrote De Materia Medica

   b. Hippocrates He established the theory of humors

3. Patient-focused care and a multidisciplinary healthcare team are essential in today's medical community. Most models of care have four contributors to a patient's supervision: physician, nurse, pharmacist, and caregiver. What are the roles of each of these contributors, and what responsibilities do they have toward the patient?

   a. physician _____
   _____

   b. nurse _____
   _____

   c. pharmacist _____
   _____

d. caregiver _____

_____

4. Contrast the work environment in a community pharmacy with that of a hospital pharmacy for a pharmacy technician. What are the perceived advantages and disadvantages? Which do you think you would prefer and why?

_____

_____

_____

_____

WEB ACTIVITIES

1. Visit the Pharmacy Museum site, at www.pharmacy.arizona.edu/about/, and take the virtual tour. Make a list of 10 things you found interesting; then answer the following questions:

   a. What were the red and green show globes used to indicate?_____

   _____

   b. Who was the famous visitor to the Owl Drug Store?_____

   _____

   c. How large is the ice cream maker? _____

   _____

   d. What is the old autoclave made of? _____

   _____

   e. What did old Jess collect from under the counter and place in a jar? _____

   _____

   f. What company produced the Materia Medica?_____

   _____

   g. What is Chill Tonic used for?_____

   _____

   h. What type of medicine was Humphrey's Specifics?_____

   _____

   i. What types of games did the pharmacy have? _____

   _____

   j. What could you win? _____

   _____

   k. What was the Lloyd continuous extraction apparatus once used for? _____

   _____

2. Type the keywords **pharmacy history** into a search engine (e.g., Google, at www.google.com). From this search you will find that numerous sites in the United States have a summary of pharmacy history. Check a Web link about pharmacy history in your state or region. Also look for sites that describe how pharmacy has evolved in Germany, Denmark, Norway, and Canada. Find two sites from these countries, and compare the key milestones in pharmacy history that are presented on all these sites and on your local or regional site. Did the development of pharmacies in the United States follow a pattern similar to that of pharmacies in other countries? Explain.

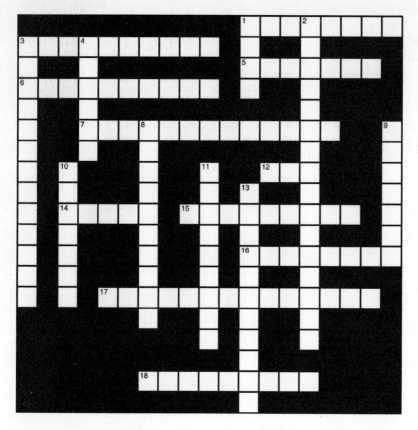

17. philosophy of care that includes ensuring positive outcomes with drug therapy

18. pharmacy that dispenses prescription medications to patients outside a hospital setting

Down

1. place where a pharmacy delivers medical supplies for patients who have been released from medical facilities

2. study of the absorption, distribution, metabolism, and elimination of drugs within the body

3. study of the release characteristics of specific drug dose forms

4. another name for a community pharmacy

8. paraprofessional who helps a licensed pharmacist carry out routine duties

9. care facility that provides specialized medical services for geriatric and disabled patients over a long period of time

10. pharmacy that prepares and distributes radioactive pharmaceuticals to treat and diagnose disease

11. list of drugs that a committee of health professionals has approved for use

13. retail pharmacy that is privately owned by the pharmacist

Across

1. pharmacy operating in an institution that provides 24-hour medical and surgical care

3. one who is licensed to prepare and dispense prescription drugs, counsel patients, and monitor response to therapy

5. type of health insurance system that focuses on reducing healthcare costs by keeping patients healthy and controlling diseases

6. another name sometimes used for a franchise pharmacy

7. pharmacy that is associated with an organized healthcare system, such as a hospital, home healthcare provider, long-term care facility, or managed-care organization

12. another name for managed care

14. group of similar pharmacies that are owned by a corporation

15. independently owned pharmacy that is a member of a chain of pharmacies

16. care facility that provides routine medical services for geriatric and disabled patients over a long period of time

Pharmacy Law, Regulations, and Standards for Technicians

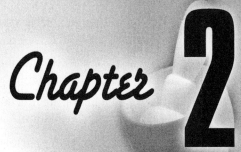

Chapter 2

COMMUNICATION AND PHARMACY PRACTICE

1. Define the following legal terms:

   a. law _____

   _____

   b. common law _____

   _____

   c. criminal law _____

   _____

   d. statutory law _____

   _____

   e. regulatory or administrative law _____

   _____

   f. ethics _____

   _____

   g. professional standards_____

   _____

2. Provide the term naming each of the following elements of law:

   a. the requirement to prove a case in a court or hearing _____

   b. the requirement to provide convincing evidence that the defendant committed the act _____

   c. failure to provide the minimum standard of care_____

   d. the legal principle that the physician is an intermediary between the drug company and the patient needing a particular medication and that the physician has the duty to provide the patient with education about the drug _____

---

e. the requirement that a case have enough evidence to support proceeding to trial _____

f. the determination that two or more causes are a factor in the negligence and personal injury to the patient_____

g. one of the functions of the pharmacist required by the Omnibus Budget Reconciliation Act of 1990 (OBRA-90) _____

h. the legal principle that an employee acts as an agent for his or her employer and the employer must then answer for the actions of the employee_____

i. a legal order to appear or to provide documents _____

3. Name each of the laws described here:

a. was the first law to require marketed drugs to be unadulterated _____
Pure Food + Drug Act of 1906

b. allows time to be added to drug patents _*Drug Price*_
*Competition + Patent-Term Restoration 1984*

c. led to the formation of the FDA _*Food, Drug + Cosmetic*_
*Act of 1938*

d. requires the pharmacist to ensure informed consent for patients and prescription drugs _*DEA*_
_____

e. prohibits reimported drugs from sale in the United States _*Prescription*_
*Drug Marketing Act of 1987*

f. divides drugs into legend and nonlegend _*Food + Drug*_
*Administration Modernization Act*

g. led to the formation of the DEA _*Comprehensive Drug*_
*Abuse Prevention + Control Act 1970*

h. requires child-resistant caps to be on most prescription drugs _____
*Poison Prevention Act of 1970*

i. provides incentives to develop drugs for rare illnesses _____
*Orphan Drug Act of 1983*

j. requires drugs to be safe and effective before they can gain FDA approval
*Kefauver-Harris Amendment of 1962*

4. Contact your state board of pharmacy for information about the legal definition of the role of the pharmacy technician; licensure, registration, and/or certification requirements; and allowable duties of pharmacy technicians in your state. Write a report detailing these.

5. Read *Accreditation Standard for Pharmacy Technician Training Programs* at the American Society of Health-System Pharmacists (ASHP) Web site (www.ashp.org). Review Practice Standard VI on technician training programs. Reflect on each objective and comment on ones you feel you have met and ones for which you need additional training or experience to practice in a hospital setting.

6. Explain what is done improperly in each of the following situations, citing relevant laws or regulations as explained in Chapter 2 of the text:

   a. A telephone call comes into the pharmacy, and the technician answers the phone. The pharmacist is very busy, and the pharmacy is understaffed. The technician takes the prescription, committing it to writing for review by the pharmacist.

   b. A pharmacy technician, working a long night shift in a hospital, takes a mild amphetamine from stock and ingests it to stay awake and to carry out his duties.

   c. A pharmacist takes a prescription over the telephone but fails to commit it to writing.

   d. A pharmacy dispenses 800 mg of mebendazole tablets in a non-child-resistant container, with a specific request from the prescribing physician or the customer.

   e. A hospital technician retrieves unused meds from a ward and then checks these to make sure that they are in good condition before returning them to stock.

7. Explain the difference between federal and state pharmacy laws, and identify which takes precedence in case of a conflict. Identify, from your state pharmacy practice act, differences between federal and state law, if any.

   _____

   _____

   _____

8. Identify the state agency responsible for inpatient drug dispensing, outpatient drug dispensing, enforcement of state-controlled substances, and enforcement of federal laws for controlled substances._____

   _____

9. Identify, in your state pharmacy practice act, legal authority for pharmacists, interns, residents, and technicians in providing pharmaceutical services.

   _____

10. Identify statements from your state pharmacy practice act relating to pharmacy and technician students and interns._____

   _____

11. Describe areas of pharmacy practice covered by (a) the Food, Drug, and Cosmetic (FDC) Act of 1938; (b) the Comprehensive Drug Abuse Prevention and Control Act of 1970 (Controlled Substances Act [CSA]); and (c) the Poison Prevention Packaging Act of 1970. _____

_____

_____

_____

_____

_____

12. List necessary components of a label for controlled substances. _____

_____

_____

13. Describe the following four schedules of controlled substances, and give two examples of each schedule:

   a. Schedule II (C-II) _____

   _____

   _____

   b. Schedule III (C-III) _____

   _____

   _____

   c. Schedule IV (C-IV) _____

   _____

   _____

   d. Schedule V (C-V) _____

   _____

   _____

14. What are refill and record-keeping requirements for hydrocodone bitartrate 10/650 and Endocet 10/650? Check the *Physician's Desk Reference (PDR)* for help answering this question. _____

_____

_____

WEB ACTIVITIES

1. Visit www.whitehousedrugpolicy.gov/ and find some of the street terms for illegal drugs and narcotics that you hear about in the news. _____

    _____

    _____

2. Visit the FDA site, at www.fda.gov, and view the information in the following options:

    a. Drugs

    b. Biologics

    c. Information for Patients

3. Visit the DEA site, at www.dea.gov.

    a. What is the latest news?_____

    _____

    _____

    b. Under Recent Cases, check and summarize the August 30, 2005, press release._____

    _____

    _____

PUZZLING TERMINOLOGY

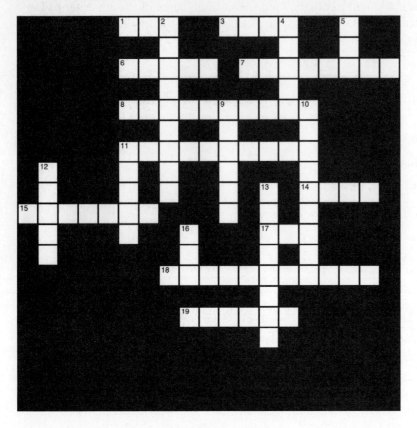

18. form of negligence in which the standard of care was not met and was a direct cause of injury

19. principle by which an employee may enter contracts on the employer's behalf

Down

2. party that files a lawsuit for the courts to decide

4. another word for brand name

5. process through which drug manufacturers formally propose that the Food and Drug Administration (FDA) approve a new pharmaceutical for sale and marketing in the United States

9. medication approved by the FDA to treat rare diseases

10. party being sued in a lawsuit

11. areas of the law that concern U.S. citizens and the wrongs they commit against one another

12. system operated by the FDA and Centers for Disease Control (CDC) that collects information on adverse events that occur after immunization

13. voluntary program run by the FDA for reporting adverse reactions with drugs, biologics, diet supplements, and medical devices

16. agency of the federal government that is responsible for ensuring the safety and efficacy of drugs prepared for the market

Across

1. agency that publishes a book containing the U.S. standards for drug formulation and dose form

3. legal term for personal injuries

6. name under which a manufacturer markets a drug

7. level of care that is usual and customary in the community

8. regulated by law owing to a potential for abuse

11. prescription containers with special lids designed to prevent children from poisoning themselves

14. organization that helps set professional standards for pharmacists

15. common name given to a drug regardless of brand name; sometimes denotes a drug that is not protected by a trademark

17. branch of the U.S. Justice Department that is responsible for regulating the sale and use of controlled substances

Drugs, Dose Forms, and Delivery Systems

Chapter 3

COMMUNICATION AND PHARMACY PRACTICE

1. Define the following terms:

   a. elixir _____

   _____

   b. legend drug _____

   _____

   c. tincture _____

   _____

2. List the advantages the given dose form has over its alternative.

   a. nitroglycerin patch chosen over nitroglycerin SL tabs _____

   _____

   _____

   b. cream over ointment _____

   _____

   _____

   c. ointment over cream _____

   _____

   _____

   d. Amoxil suspension over Amoxil capsules _____

   _____

   _____

   e. Isordil chewable tablets over Isordil oral tablets _____

   _____

   _____

f. Cardizem long-acting (LA) tablets over Cardizem sustained-release (SR) capsules_____

_____

_____

g. topical hydrocortisone cream over oral steroid tablets _____

_____

_____

h. nasal aerosol over nasal aqueous spray_____

_____

_____

i. oral albuterol over inhaled albuterol _____

_____

_____

j. rectal Dulcolax over oral Dulcolax _____

_____

_____

3. Many over-the-counter (OTC) medications are commonly found in a household.

a. Make a list of the OTC items in your home. _____

_____

_____

_____

b. What dose forms are represented? _____

_____

_____

_____

c. Describe why certain dose forms are selected by the consumer._____

_____

_____

_____

WEB ACTIVITIES

1. Visit the Web site for GlaxoSmithKline, at www.gsk.com, or one of the many sites maintained by a pharmaceutical manufacturer. Search for products that the manufacturer provides, and the various dose forms in which individual drugs are available. Prepare a list of 10 items that are available in more than one dose form.

    _____   _____

    _____   _____

    _____   _____

    _____   _____

    _____   _____

2. Visit www.claritin.com.

    a. Under Allergy Authority, check major allergens in your region and list them here._____

    _____

    b. What are the different OTC dose forms available? _____

    _____

    c. What are the advantages of each dose form? _____

    _____

    _____

Puzzle A

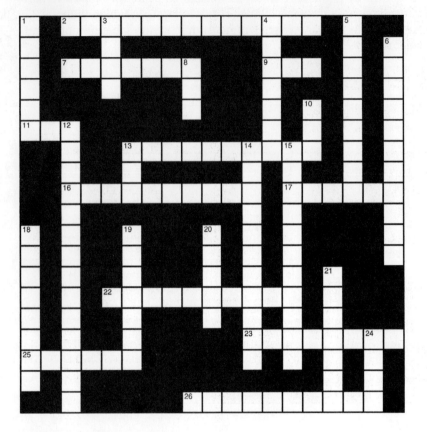

Across

2. genetic engineering technique used for creating monoclonal antibodies (MAbs)

7. vehicle that makes up the greater part of a solution

9. infusion device used by a patient to deliver small doses of medication for chronic pain

11. important component of genetic code that arranges amino acids into proteins

13. drugs used to analyze the cause of diseases

16. dose form that delivers medication from the mouth into the lungs, or from the nostril into the sinuses

17. solid dose form produced by compression and containing one or more active ingredients

22. another word for drug

23. dispersion of a liquid in another liquid

25. in a drug, ingredient that produces the desired therapeutic effect

26. sterile solution, with or without medication, that is injected through the skin

Down

1. insert that administers active medication directly into the eye

3. syringe used to wash out the eyes or ears with liquid

4. dose form placed under the skin to deliver the active ingredient slowly

5. dispersion containing ultra-fine particles

6. solid formulation for administering drugs through a body orifice such as the rectum

8. method of delivering medication through the skin, like a patch

10. unique number assigned to a product to identify the manufacturer or distributor, drug, and packaging size and type

12. drugs used to kill cancer cells

13. helix-shaped molecule that carries the genetic code

14. drug that is artificially created

15. drug delivery system that administers medications or fluids directly into a vein

18. property of a medication that is determined by its dose form

19. sweet-tasting formulation that allows medication to be absorbed in the mouth

20. cosmetically acceptable oil-in-water (O/W) emulsion for use on the skin

21. solid or semisolid, medicated or nonmedicated preparation that adheres to the skin

24. syringes without needles, used to administer medications into the mouths of patients who are unable to swallow tablets or capsules

Puzzle B

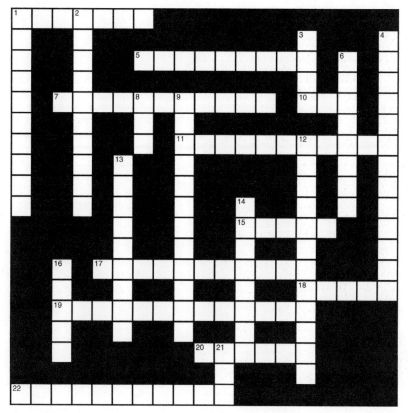

Across

1. dose form containing powder, liquid, or granules in a gelatin covering

5. device used to deliver medication in a fine mist deep into the lungs

7. type of DNA constructed of segments taken from different sources

10. dispersion containing fine particles for topical use on the skin

11. drug that prevents, cures, diagnoses, or relieves symptoms of a disease

15. inactive chemicals that are added to active ingredients to improve drug formulations

17. drug that kills bacteria, fungi, virus, or even normal or cancer cells

18. dose form that emits a fine dispersion of liquid, solid, or gaseous material

19. drugs that contain both natural and synthetic components

20. liquid for topical application, containing insoluble dispersed solids or immiscible liquids

22. medications formed by using very small dilutions of natural drugs claimed to stimulate the immune system

Down

1. dose form that regulates the rate at which a medication is released into the body

2. dispersion of a solid in a liquid

3. medical substance or remedy used to change the way a living organism functions

4. science that combines biology, chemistry, and immunology to produce synthetic, unique drugs with specific therapeutic effects

6. aqueous, alcoholic, or hydroalcoholic dose form

8. single-cell antibody that is produced in a laboratory to fight cancer and diagnose conditions such as pregnancy and syphilis

9. drug delivery system that is placed into the uterus

12. gas-releasing, as in granular salts that bubble and dispense active ingredients when placed in water

13. drug that is artificially created in imitation of naturally occurring substances

14. semisolid emulsion for topical use on the skin

16. water-in-oil (W/O) emulsion containing more solid material than ointments

21. drug sold without a prescription

Routes of Drug Administration

Chapter 4

COMMUNICATION AND PHARMACY PRACTICE

1. Define the following terms:

    a. compliance _____

    _____

    b. conjunctival _____

    _____

    c. ophthalmic _____

    _____

    d. rectal _____

    _____

    e. transdermal _____

    _____

    f. first-pass effect _____

    _____

    g. infusion _____

    _____

    h. otic _____

    _____

2. Describe the site at which the following injections are administered:

    a. intradermal (ID) _____

    b. intramuscular (IM) _____

    c. intravenous (IV) _____

    d. subcutaneous _____

3. A patient has just brought in a prescription for Compazine suppositories, and would like to have the prescription filled for Compazine capsules instead. He does not like the idea of using rectal suppositories.

a. Are the two dose forms used for the same thing? _____

_____

b. What are the advantages of the suppository form that the patient might not have considered? How will the pharmacist explain this to the patient?

_____

_____

_____

4. What verb should be used at the beginning of the sentence when giving instructions on the prescription label or medication order for the following routes?

a. oral _____

b. intramuscular (IM) _____

c. topical _____

d. buccal _____

e. vaginal _____

f. rectal _____

g. ophthalmic _____

h. otic _____

i. intranasal _____

j. intrarespiratory _____

WEB ACTIVITIES

1. Visit the Web site for the periodical *Drug Topics,* at www.drugtopics.com, and read a recent article that interests you. Summarize it and turn in a report for evaluation.

2. Visit www.uspharmacist.com, the Web site for the periodical *U.S. Pharmacist,* and read a recent article that interests you. Summarize it and turn in a report for evaluation.

PUZZLING TERMINOLOGY

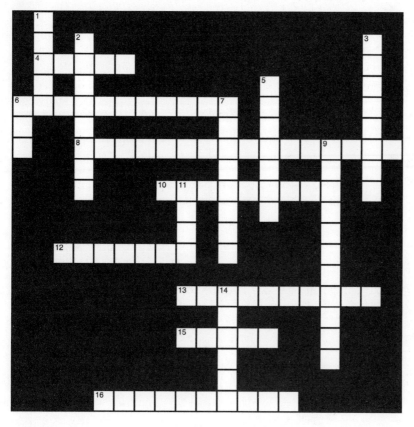

15. site-specific application of a drug

16. study of the poisonous effects of drugs or substances in the body

Down

1. size of dose that must be given to counteract the first-pass effect of some drugs

2. length of time that a drug gives the desired response or is at the therapeutic level

3. administration of a drug by insertion into the urethra

5. administration of a drug to the skin or a mucous membrane

6. device used to administer a drug in the form of compressed gas through inhalation into the lungs

7. application of a drug by absorption into the bloodstream

9. desired pharmacological action of a drug on the body

11. administration of a drug into the gastrointestinal (GI) tract through swallowing

14. administration in which a drug is placed between the gums and the inner lining of the cheek

Across

4. way of getting a drug onto or into the body

6. inactive drugs that remain after the liver breaks down active drugs

8. administration of a drug by inhalation into the lungs

10. occurs when the body requires higher doses of a drug to produce the same therapeutic effect

12. administration of a drug by application into the vagina

13. administration of a drug through placement under the tongue

Basic Pharmaceutical Measurements and Calculations

Chapter **5**

MATHEMATICS REVIEW

Metric System

1. Convert the following amounts:

    a. 3.8 mg = _____ mcg

    b. 840 mg = _____ g

    c. 1225 mg = _____ g

    d. 0.125 mg = _____ mcg

2. Convert the following amounts:

    a. 240 mL = _____ L

    b. 0.5 L = _____ mL

    c. 320 mL = _____ L

    d. 0.034 L = _____ mL

3. Convert the following amounts:

    a. 30 mL = _____ L

    b. 250 mg = _____ g

    c. 0.75 mg = _____ mcg

    d. 1.62 g = _____ mg

4. You need to dispense 500 mg of a drug. It is available in a 1 g tablet. What will you dispense?

5. You need to prepare 1.8 g of a drug available as 500 mg/2 mL. What will you prepare?

6. How many milligrams are in 7 mL of a 35 mg/10 mL drug?

7. How many grams are in 3 mL of a 1.25 g/15 mL drug?

8. How many 125 mg tablets will be needed to provide a patient with a 6 g dose?

Metric System Conversions

1. Convert the following amounts:

   a. 520 mg = _____ gr

   b. 1131 mg = _____ gr

   c. 24 mg = _____ gr

   d. 250 mg = _____ gr

2. Convert the following amounts:

   a. 10 gr = _____ mg

   b. 3 gr = _____ mg

   c. 5 gr = _____ mg

   d. 18 gr = _____ g

3. How many pounds do the following patients weigh?

   a. 14 kg = _____ lb

   b. 106 kg = _____ lb

   c. 8.4 kg = _____ lb

   d. 0.94 kg = _____ lb

4. How many kilograms do the following patients weigh?

   a. 84 lb = _____ kg

   b. 138 lb = _____ kg

   c. 194 lb = _____ kg

   d. 218 lb = _____ kg

5. Convert the following amounts:

   a. 8 fl oz = _____ mL

   b. 4 tsp = _____ mL

   c. 6 tbsp = _____ mL

   d. 14 fl oz = _____ mL

6. Convert the following amounts:

   a. 6 fl oz = _____ mL

   b. 2 fl oz = _____ mL

   c. 1.4 pt = _____ mL

   d. 0.5 fl oz = _____ mL

7. Convert the following amounts:

   a. 11 oz = _____ g

   b. 200 g = _____ oz

   c. 39 g = _____ oz

   d. 894 g = _____ oz

8. Convert the following amounts:

   a. 12 gr = _____ mg

   b. 0.4 gr = _____ mg

   c. 39 mL = _____ fl oz

   d. 23 gr = _____ g

9. If 250 mg are in 5 mL, how many grams are in 8 fl oz?

10. If 50 mg are in 50 mL, how many milligrams are in 6 tsp?

11. What is the total amount of drug in milligrams given if a patient takes ½ tsp of a 1 g/5 mL suspension?

12. What is the amount of drug in a 2 tsp dose of a 125 mg/5 mL antibiotic suspension?

13. A patient who weighs 89 lb is to get a dose of 0.35 mg/kg. How many milligrams will that be?

14. A patient who weighs 124 kg is to get a dose of 10 mg/lb daily. The dose should be taken three times a day (tid). How much is each dose?

15. You are to prepare 350 mg of a medication from a 2 gr/3 mL solution. How much will you need?

16. How many days will 150 mL last a patient if the order is to take 1 fluidram tid?

17. How long will 12 fl oz last if the patient uses ½ tbsp tid and at bedtime (hs)?

18. How many 325 mg aspirin tablets should a patient take if the recommended dose is 5 gr qAM?

19. You need to prepare 450 mg of a medication available as 1.5 g/2 tbsp dose. How many drams is this?

20. You are to prepare a 1 tsp dose of a drug available as 800 mg/fl oz. How many milligrams is the dose?

Fractions and Decimals

1. Write the following Arabic numerals as Roman numerals:

   a. 27 = _____

   b. 94 = _____

   c. 306 = _____

   d. 1300 = _____

2. Write the following Roman numerals as Arabic numerals:

   a. VII = _____

   b. XXVI = _____

   c. XCII = _____

   d. CCVII = _____

3. Convert the following fractions to decimals:

   a. $\frac{3}{4}$ = _____

   b. $\frac{5}{16}$ = _____

   c. $\frac{8}{20}$ = _____

   d. $5\frac{2}{7}$ = _____

4. Convert the following decimals to fractions:

   a. 0.5 = _____

   b. 0.125 = _____

   c. 1.8 = _____

   d. 0.333 = _____

5. Calculate the following amounts:

   a. 0.45×0.9 = _____

   b. $\frac{1}{2} + \frac{5}{6}$ = _____

   c. $\frac{3}{8} - \frac{1}{16}$ = _____

   d. $0.75 \times \frac{1}{2}$ = _____

6. Circle the *largest* number in each of the following sets:

   a. 8.4   8.14   8.04

   b. 6.3   6.03   6.93

   c. 0.08   0.80   0.087

   d. 1.36   1.06   1.63

7. Circle the *smallest* number in each of the following sets:

   a. 3.40   3.04   3.08

   b. 0.931   0.932   0.909

   c. 3.11   0.311   3.04

   d. 0.134   0.043   0.143

8. Convert each of the following fractions to a mixed number:

   a. $\frac{18}{4}$ = _____

   b. $\frac{26}{3}$ = _____

   c. $\frac{4}{3}$ = _____

   d. $\frac{66}{8}$ = _____

9. Convert each of the following fractions to a decimal:

   a. $\frac{19}{3}$ = _____

   b. $\frac{3}{8}$ = _____

   c. $\frac{16}{7}$ = _____

   d. $\frac{1}{8}$ = _____

10. Convert each of the following decimals to a fraction:

    a. 0.125 = _____

    b. 0.67 = _____

    c. 1.33 = _____

    d. 0.75 = _____

Ratios, Proportions, and Percents

1. Convert the following ratios to fractions, and then reduce:

   a. 6:8

   b. 12:30

   c. 3:6

   d. 2:42

2. Solve the following equations for *x:*

   a. $x:4 = 3:12$

   b. $x:16 = 5:30$

   c. $x:10 = 125:5$

   d. $x:375 = 2:500$

3. Calculate the following amounts:

   a. 18% of 150 = _____

   b. 85% of 620 = _____

   c. 0.9% of 1000 = _____

   d. 5% of 50 = _____

4. Convert the following ratios to percents:

   a. 4:10 = _____

   b. 3:8 = _____

   c. 1:32 = _____

   d. 1:500 = _____

5. Fill in the missing values in the following table:

Fraction	Decimal	Ratio	Percent
$\frac{1}{2}$	a. _____	b. _____	c. _____
d. _____	e. _____	7:4	f. _____
g. _____	0.75	h. _____	i. _____
j. _____	k. _____	l. _____	10%
$\frac{9}{5}$	m. _____	n. _____	o. _____

6. Fill in the missing values in the following table:

Fraction	Decimal	Ratio	Percent
$\frac{5}{8}$	a. _____	b. _____	c. _____
d. _____	e. _____	2:3	f. _____
g. _____	1.90	h. _____	i. _____
j. _____	k. _____	l. _____	0.5%
$\frac{1}{3}$	m. _____	n. _____	o. _____

7. You are to prepare 275 mg of a drug that is available as 800 mg/5 mL. What volume of solution will you prepare?

8. You need to prepare a 0.375 mg dose. You have 0.125 mg and 0.25 mg tablets. How many tablets of each strength will you prepare?

9. You need to prepare a 100 mg dose for intramuscular (IM) injection. What volume of a 200 mg/mL solution will you prepare?

10. You need to prepare 150 mg of a solution available as 80 mg/15 mL. What will you prepare?

Pharmaceutical Solutions

1. You are to reconstitute a drug available in a 250 mg dry powder form by adding 4.6 mL diluent. The final concentration is to be 50 mg/mL.

   a. What is the powder volume?

   _____

   b. How many milliliters would be prepared for a 125 mg dose?

   _____

2. You are to reconstitute 3 g of a drug available in a dry powder form by adding a diluent. The powder volume is 0.5 mL.

    a. How much diluent will you add if the desired concentration is 600 mg/2 mL?

    _____

    b. How many milligrams of drug will be in 1.4 mL of the prepared product?

    _____

3. How many milliliters are needed to prepare a 100 mg dose if the concentration is 500 mg in 4 mL after the diluent is added?

4. If an order is received to make 240 mL of a 1% solution with water and a 40% stock solution, how much of each is needed?

5. If an order is received to make 30 mL of a 0.25% solution with water and a 10% stock dilution, how much of each is needed?

6. The order says to make 60 g of a 3% cream. You have 1% and 10% to mix together. How much of each will you use?

7. The order says to make 480 mL of 50% alcohol solution. You have 70% and 30% to mix together. How much of each will you use?

8. If an order is received to make 1 lb of a 15% ointment and you have a 40% and a 10% ointment, how many grams will you use of each?

PUZZLING TERMINOLOGY

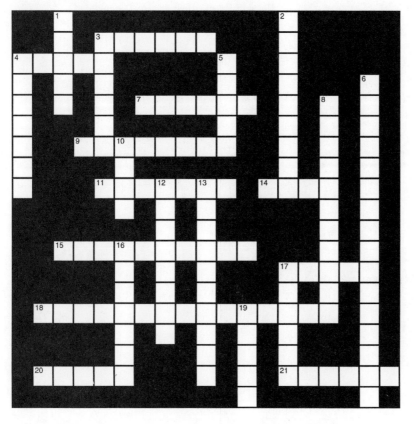

Down

1. mathematical expression comparing two amounts or numbers

2. number on the top part of a fraction

3. fraction with a value less than 1

4. zero that is placed in the one's place in a decimal number that is less than zero

5. system for expressing numbers using units such as I, V, X, ss, i, v, x, l, c, d, and m

6. another name for a mixed number

8. number on the bottom part of a fraction

10. measurement of extension in space in two dimensions

12. fraction with a value greater than 1

13. concentration created by compounding different solutions with the same active ingredient in differing strengths

16. part of 100

17. measurement system based on subdivisions and multiples of 10

19. number consisting of an integer and a fraction

Across

3. volume occupied by a dry medication in a sterile vial

4. base metric unit used for measuring volume

7. measurement of extension in space in three dimensions

9. portion of a whole that is represented as a ratio

11. number that can be written in decimal notation using the integers 0 through 9 and a point (.)

14. base metric unit used for measuring weight

15. mathematical expression comparing two ratios that have the same value

17. base metric unit used for measuring length

18. equivalent to 1 mL

20. smallest common denominator

21. denominator shared by two or more fractions

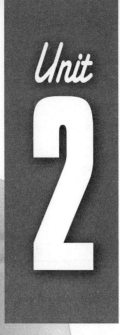

Unit 2

Community Pharmacy

Dispensing Medications in the Community Pharmacy

Chapter 6

COMMUNICATION AND PHARMACY PRACTICE

If necessary, use Appendix A in the textbook to answer questions 1 to 3.

1. Write out instructions using lay terms for the following orders. Include a verb and the route when known.

   a. 1 tab po every other day_____

   b. 1 R q6h prn N&V_____

   c. 41 units subcutaneous qAM_____

   d. 3 cap po hs _____

   e. 5 gr po qAM _____

   f. 1 cap po qPM _____

   g. ½ tab po tid x 20d_____

   h. apply ung bid _____

   i. 5 mL po qAM _____

   j. 3 gtt au hs x 3d _____

2. Write out instructions using lay terms for the following orders. Include a verb and the route when known.

   a. 1 cap po bid _____

   b. 1 cap po qAM pc _____

   c. 1 tab tid po till gone _____

   d. 2 tsp po tid x 10d_____

   e. 4 tab stat, 2 in 6h _____

   f. ½ tsp po q4–6h _____

   g. 1–2 tab po q3–4h prn pain_____

   h. 3 gtt AD bid _____

   i. apply to lips 5x daily_____

   j. 1 app vag hs x 7d _____

---

3. Write out instructions using lay terms for the following orders. Include a verb and the route when known.

    a. 1 cap po q hs, 2 cap qAM _____

    b. 1 tab po q6h prn _____

    c. 1 cap qid po x 7d_____

    d. 1 tab po ac _____

    e. 1 gtt ou qAM _____

    f. 1 supp R prn N&V & hs _____

    g. 4 gtt as prn pain_____

    h. apply hs_____

    i. apply ut dict _____

    j. apply qid leg_____

4. Read the following prescriptions and prepare labels for them. In addition, look up which auxiliary labels would be applied to the prescription vials.

Auxiliary Label

a.
    ℞ Tobrex opth sol
    3 gtt OS tid x 7 days
    Disp 10 mL

Paragon Pharmacy	AP 1111111
670 Main Street	220-555-3245
Anytown, USA	
Patient: _____	Prescriber: _____
Drug: _____	
Date: _____	Refills: _____

_____

_____

_____

_____

b.
    ℞ Calan SR 240 mg
    take 1 po qAM
    #90

Paragon Pharmacy	AP 1111111
670 Main Street	220-555-3245
Anytown, USA	
Patient: _____	Prescriber: _____
Drug: _____	
Date: _____	Refills: _____

_____

_____

_____

_____

c.   R$_X$ Coumadin 2 mg
take 1 tab hs
#10

Paragon Pharmacy   AP 1111111
670 Main Street   220-555-3245
Anytown, USA

Patient: _____   Prescriber: _____

Drug: _____

Date: _____   Refills: _____

d.   R$_X$ Zoloft 50 mg
1½ tab hs
#45

Paragon Pharmacy   AP 1111111
670 Main Street   220-555-3245
Anytown, USA

Patient: _____   Prescriber: _____

Drug: _____

Date: _____   Refills: _____

e.   R$_X$ Lasix 40 mg
1 qAM c̄ potassium
#30

Paragon Pharmacy   AP 1111111
670 Main Street   220-555-3245
Anytown, USA

Patient: _____   Prescriber: _____

Drug: _____

Date: _____   Refills: _____

Name _____   **Date** _____   • *Chapter 6*   **39**

f. R_X Glucotrol 500 mg
      1 ac po
      #90

Paragon Pharmacy	AP 1111111
670 Main Street	220-555-3245
Anytown, USA	
Patient: _____	Prescriber: _____
Drug: _____	
Date: _____	Refills: _____

_____

_____

_____

_____

g. R_X Naprosyn 500 mg
      Sig: 1 bid c̄ food
      #60

Paragon Pharmacy	AP 1111111
670 Main Street	220-555-3245
Anytown, USA	
Patient: _____	Prescriber: _____
Drug: _____	
Date: _____	Refills: _____

_____

_____

_____

_____

h. R_X amoxicillin 250 mg/5 mL
      one tsp tid
      disp 150 mL

Paragon Pharmacy	AP 1111111
670 Main Street	220-555-3245
Anytown, USA	
Patient: _____	Prescriber: _____
Drug: _____	
Date: _____	Refills: _____

_____

_____

_____

_____

i. R_X Toradol 10 mg
one tab q8h prn
Disp: 20 tabs

Paragon Pharmacy	AP 1111111
670 Main Street	220-555-3245
Anytown, USA	
Patient: _____	Prescriber: _____

_____

_____

_____

_____

Drug: _____

Date: _____   Refills: _____

j. R_X Atrovent MDI
use 2 puffs bid
Disp #1

Paragon Pharmacy	AP 1111111
670 Main Street	220-555-3245
Anytown, USA	
Patient: _____	Prescriber: _____

_____

_____

_____

_____

Drug: _____

Date: _____   Refills: _____

WEB ACTIVITIES

1.   Visit the Pharmex Web site, at www.pharmex.com, and look at the various options available to the user.

   a.   For what is the company well known?_____

   _____

   _____

   b.   Take a look at the various labels available, and make a list of the 10 labels (besides the top sellers) that you think would be particularly useful. State on what type of product they would be used.

   _____

   _____

   _____

_____

_____

_____

_____

_____

_____

2. Visit the Apothecary Products Web site, at www.apothecaryproducts.com, and look at the on-line catalog.

   a. What types of products does this company offer for resale? _____

   _____

   _____

   b. What types of promotional products can be purchased? _____

   _____

   _____

   _____

   c. If you had a budget of $1,000.00, what promotional items would you order to promote your pharmacy? _____

   _____

   _____

   _____

IN THE LAB

To answer the following questions, you will need to use the appropriate drug reference materials.

1. Ms. Mary Lawson has the following prescriptions currently on file at The Corner Drug Store:

Prescription No.	Medication	Directions	Date Dispensed	Refills
12345	Ortho-Novum 7/7/7	one tab daily	12/27/XX	6
12346	Pepcid 20 mg	one tab daily	1/3/XX	4
12347	Darvocet-N 100	one tab q4–6h prn	4/16/XX	2

a. Ms. Lawson has brought in a new prescription for Ery-Tab 333. Are there potential interactions with any of her current medications? If so, please describe them. _____

_____

_____

b. According to the file, one of the prescriptions Ms. Lawson is taking is Darvocet-N 100.

    1) What is this medication? _____

       _____

    2) What schedule is it? _____

       _____

    3) What is the maximum recommended dose of each ingredient per day? _____

       _____

c. According to the file, one of the prescriptions Ms. Lawson is taking is Pepcid 20 mg.

    1) What class of medication is Pepcid? _____

       _____

    2) What are some other medications in this class? _____

       _____

       _____

    3) Are there any over-the-counter (OTC) products in this class? If so, name them. _____

       _____

       _____

2. Consumers are turning increasingly to products they can purchase at will and can self-administer for their health problems. A number of factors affect this change. At the forefront are economic trends, increased cost of physician visits, rising cost of prescription medications, and changes in insurance coverage.

    Although OTC medications may be purchased without a prescription, the active ingredients generally are the same as those found in higher-strength prescription versions. The Food and Drug Administration (FDA) will approve an OTC preparation when the agency is assured the dose strength is beneficial and yet not likely to cause harm to the general public when taken as directed.

    Pharmacists are devoting a greater amount of their time to recommending OTC products to their customers. The inventory and counseling responsibilities of OTC products are being shifted to the pharmacy technician, and these products will become an increasingly important part of the pharmacy technician's work.

    In this exercise you will review the medication categories and provide the following information for each product. (*Caution:* Some products change formulation or may be restricted for OTC sales in some states.)

        AI: active ingredient or ingredients
        DA: drug action (how it works, what it does)
        IU: indication for use (what condition is product used for)

Allergy

Chlor-Trimeton (liquid)

AI: _____

DA: _____

IU: _____

Benadryl Allergy/Cold
(capsules/tablets)

AI: _____

DA: _____

IU: _____

Neo-Synephrine (liquid/spray)

AI: _____

DA: _____

IU: _____

Cold/Cough

Comtrex, adult cold product
(tablets)

AI: _____

DA: _____

IU: _____

Dimetapp Children's
Cold and Cough

AI: _____

DA: _____

IU: _____

TheraFlu

AI: _____

DA: _____

IU: _____

Sudafed (tablets)

AI: _____

DA: _____

IU: _____

Chloraseptic (spray)

AI: _____

DA: _____

IU: _____

Gastrointestinal

Maalox (liquid)

AI: _____

DA: _____

IU: _____

Mylanta (gel capsules)

AI: _____

DA: _____

IU: _____

Gas-X   AI: _____   • _____

                               DA: _____

                               IU: _____

Imodium A-D   AI: _____

                               DA: _____

                               IU: _____

Metamucil   AI: _____

                               DA: _____

                               IU: _____

Dulcolax   AI: _____

                               DA: _____

                               IU: _____

Oral Care

Phos-Flur   AI: _____

                               DA: _____

                               IU: _____

Pain Reliever

Advil (tablets)   AI: _____

                               DA: _____

                               IU: _____

Myoflex   AI: _____

                               DA: _____

                               IU: _____

Excedrin (tablets)   AI: _____

                               DA: _____

                               IU: _____

Tylenol (drops)   AI: _____

                               DA: _____

                               IU: _____

Personal Care

Nix (cream rinse)   AI: _____

                               DA: _____

                               IU: _____

Xero-Lube

AI: _____

DA: _____

IU: _____

Visine (eyedrops)

AI: _____

DA: _____

IU: _____

Preparation H (cream)

AI: _____

DA: _____

IU: _____

Sominex

AI: _____

DA: _____

IU: _____

Monistat 7 (vaginal cream)

AI: _____

DA: _____

IU: _____

Replens (liquid)

AI: _____

DA: _____

IU: _____

Skin Care

Oxy 10 (cream)

AI: _____

DA: _____

IU: _____

Persa-Gel (gel)

AI: _____

DA: _____

IU: _____

Cortaid (cream)

AI: _____

DA: _____

IU: _____

Tinactin (spray)

AI: _____

DA: _____

IU: _____

Lubriderm (lotion)

AI: _____

DA: _____

IU: _____

Micatin (cream)   AI: _____

                         DA: _____

                         IU: _____

Neosporin (ointment)   AI: _____

                         DA: _____

                         IU: _____

4. Being able to quickly scan incoming prescriptions for completeness and missing information is a skill that is learned from reading many prescriptions. Read the following prescriptions, and state what type of information is missing on each:

Missing Information

a.

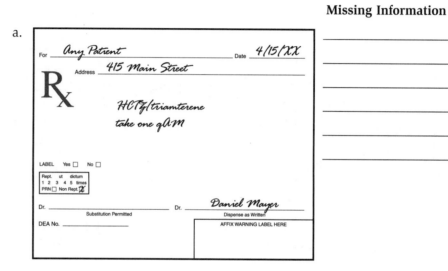

_____

_____

_____

_____

_____

_____

b.

_____

_____

_____

_____

_____

_____

c.

For _Any Patient_   Date _4/15/XX_

Address _415 Main Street_

R_X

Allegra
one tablet bid
#60

LABEL   Yes ☐   No ☐

Rept.   ut   dictum
1   2   3   4   5   times
PRN ☒ Non Rept. ☐

Dr. _____
Substitution Permitted

Dr. _____ _James Russell_
Dispense as Written

DEA No. _____

AFFIX WARNING LABEL HERE

_____
_____
_____
_____
_____
_____

d.

For _Any Patient_   Date _4/15/XX_

Address _415 Main Street_

R_X

sulfasalazine 500 mg
take 1 tid
#90

LABEL   Yes ☐   No ☐

Rept.   ut   dictum
1 ② 3   4   5   times
PRN ☐ Non Rept. ☐

Dr. _____
Substitution Permitted

Dr. _____
Dispense as Written

DEA No. _____

AFFIX WARNING LABEL HERE

_____
_____
_____
_____
_____

e.

For _Any Patient_   Date _4/15/XX_

Address _415 Main Street_

R_X

Elavil
1 hs
#30

LABEL   Yes ☐   No ☐

Rept.   ut   dictum
1   2   3 ④ 5   times
PRN ☐ Non Rept. ☐

Dr. _____
Substitution Permitted

Dr. _____ _Pamela Davis_
Dispense as Written

DEA No. _____

AFFIX WARNING LABEL HERE

_____
_____
_____
_____
_____
_____

f.

For _Any Patient_   Date _4/15/XX_

R_X

Address _415 Main Street_

     Glucotrol

     1 tab ac

LABEL   Yes ☐   No ☐

Rept.   ut   dictum
① 2 3 4 5 times
PRN ☐   Non Rept. ☐

Dr. _____   Dr. _Alex Barnwell_

Substitution Permitted   Dispense as Written

DEA No. _____

AFFIX WARNING LABEL HERE

_____
_____
_____
_____
_____
_____
_____

g.

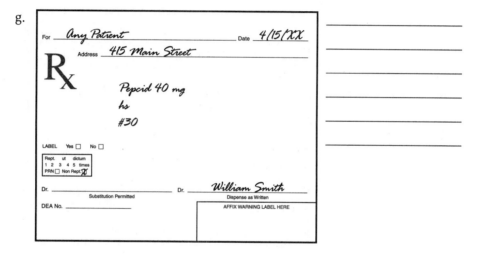

For _Any Patient_   Date _4/15/XX_

R_X

Address _415 Main Street_

     Pepcid 40 mg

     hs

     #30

LABEL   Yes ☐   No ☐

Rept.   ut   dictum
1 2 3 4 5 times
PRN ☐   Non Rept. ☒

Dr. _____   Dr. _William Smith_

Substitution Permitted   Dispense as Written

DEA No. _____

AFFIX WARNING LABEL HERE

_____
_____
_____
_____
_____
_____

h.

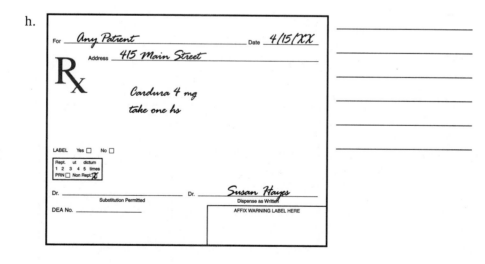

For _Any Patient_   Date _4/15/XX_

R_X

Address _415 Main Street_

     Cardura 4 mg

     take one hs

LABEL   Yes ☐   No ☐

Rept.   ut   dictum
1 2 3 4 5 times
PRN ☐   Non Rept. ☒

Dr. _____   Dr. _Susan Hayes_

Substitution Permitted   Dispense as Written

DEA No. _____

AFFIX WARNING LABEL HERE

_____
_____
_____
_____
_____
_____

i.

For _Any Patient_   Date _4/15/XX_

Address _415 Main Street_

R_X

     Zovirax 800 mg
     #50

LABEL   Yes ☐   No ☐

Rept.   ut   dictum
1   2   3   4   5   times
PRN ☐ Non Rept. ☒

Dr. _____   Dr. _Matthew Berger_
   Substitution Permitted   Dispense as Written

DEA No. _____   AFFIX WARNING LABEL HERE

_____

_____

_____

_____

_____

j.

For _Any Patient_   Date _4/15/XX_

Address _415 Main Street_

R_X

     Synthroid
     take 1 qAM
     #60

LABEL   Yes ☐   No ☐

Rept.   ut   dictum
1   2   3   4   5   times
PRN ☐ Non Rept. ☒

Dr. _____   Dr. _Andrew Rice_
   Substitution Permitted   Dispense as Written

DEA No. _____   AFFIX WARNING LABEL HERE

_____

_____

_____

_____

_____

5. Read the following prescriptions and state what type of information is missing or is incorrect on each:

Missing or Incorrect Information

a.

MT. HOPE MEDICAL PARK
MY TOWN, USA   555-3591

_____   DEA # _____
PT. NAME _Larry Walker_   DATE _1/21/XX_
ADDRESS _____

_____

R_X Tylox
     one q4–6h prn pain
     #30

REFILLS _____ TIMES (NO REFILL UNLESS INDICATED)

_____ M.D.   _____ M.D.
  DISPENSE AS WRITTEN   SUBSTITUTE PERMITTED

_____

_____

_____

_____

_____

_____

b.

MT. HOPE MEDICAL PARK
MY TOWN, USA   555-3591

#_____   DEA # _MJ12345678_
PT. NAME__Nancy Cruth_____ DATE _____
ADDRESS _____
_____

℞   Demerol 50 mg tablets
one daily
#45

REFILLS _2_ TIMES (NO REFILL UNLESS INDICATED)
_____ M.D. ___M. Johnson_____ M.D.
DISPENSE AS WRITTEN   SUBSTITUTE PERMITTED

_____
_____
_____
_____
_____
_____

c.

MT. HOPE MEDICAL PARK
MY TOWN, USA   555-3591

#_____   DEA # _____
PT. NAME__David Marsh_____ DATE _____
ADDRESS _____
_____

℞   Zantac 150 mg
1 q8h

REFILLS _3_ TIMES (NO REFILL UNLESS INDICATED)
_____ M.D. ___D. White_____ M.D.
DISPENSE AS WRITTEN   SUBSTITUTE PERMITTED

_____
_____
_____
_____
_____
_____

d.

MT. HOPE MEDICAL PARK
MY TOWN, USA   555-3591

#_____   DEA # _____
PT. NAME__David Marsh_____ DATE _____
ADDRESS _____
_____

℞   Trimox 500 mg
1 cap q8h

REFILLS _4_ TIMES (NO REFILL UNLESS INDICATED)
_____ M.D. ___D. White_____ M.D.
DISPENSE AS WRITTEN   SUBSTITUTE PERMITTED

_____
_____
_____
_____
_____
_____

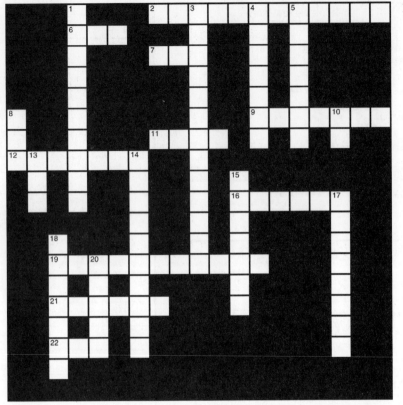

1. product used to treat common symptoms of illness or to maintain health, and sold without a prescription

3. having identical active ingredients or similar bioavailability characteristics, and producing the same effect

4. part of the patient profile that protects the pharmacy when a patient does not disclose all relevant information

5. record kept by the pharmacy that lists a patient's identifying information, insurance information, medical history, prescription history, and prescription preferences

8. number issued to a physician authorizing him or her to prescribe certain controlled substances

10. part of the prescription that means "take"

13. abbreviation indicating that the prescribed drug is not to be replaced with a generic version

14. type of prescription that is replacing written prescriptions, especially owing to the increasing use of pocket digital assistants (PDAs) by physicians

15. part of the patient profile that lists existing conditions as well as known allergies and adverse drug reactions the patient has experienced

17. type of warning required on Schedule II, III, IV, and V drugs

18. part of the patient profile that includes information about prescription drug insurance

20. part of the prescription that indicates the directions for the patient to follow

Across

2. part of the prescription that lists compounding or packaging instructions, labeling instructions, refill information, and information about the appropriateness of dispensing drug equivalencies

6. term used to describe a fixed number of dose units in a drug stock container, usually a 1-month's supply, or 30 tablets or capsules

7. abbreviation indicating that the pharmacist must dispense only the brand name version of a drug

9. state of heightened sensitivity as a result of exposure to a particular substance

11. single dose of a medication, usually heat-sealed or in a blister pack

12. negative consequence to a patient from taking a particular drug

16. information sheet required by the Food and Drug Administration (FDA) and provided by a drug manufacturer that includes the product's indication and uses, dose, contraindications and warnings, as well as side effects and adverse reactions

19. part of the prescription that lists the medication or medications prescribed, including the drug names, strengths, and amounts

21. another name for prescription drugs

22. abbreviation indicating that the patient is unaware of any allergies to medications

The Business of Community Pharmacy

Chapter 7

COMMUNICATION AND PHARMACY PRACTICE

1. How often are inventories taken for controlled substances? _____
   _____

2. Explain security requirements for controlled substance storage. _____
   _____

3. Explain distribution and record keeping for controlled substances. (Refer to Chapters 2 and 7 in answering this question.) _____
   _____

4. Visit a local community pharmacy, either locally or on the Internet.

   a. Select three common drugs that are available as a brand and a generic, and compare prices of brand versus generic. _____
      _____
      _____
      _____

   b. Identify four common insurers for prescription drugs. Select one insurer, visit its Web site, and determine its copay and formulary structure. Compare your findings with those of other students in the class.

5. Complete one or both of these tasks:

   a. Ask several older patients, including family members or friends, what their experience has been with the Medicare Part D drug insurance program. If they have questions about the program, try to answer them.

   b. List some helpful resources (Web sites, publications, and so on) regarding the Medicare Part D drug insurance program.

BUSINESS MATHEMATICS

1. Mark the following prices up 24%:

   a. $8.24 _____

   b. $283.40 _____

   c. $500.00 _____

   d. $16.90 _____

2. Mark the following prices up 8% plus $3.00:

   a. $12.50 _____

   b. $29.40 _____

   c. $106.94 _____

   d. $418.05 _____

3. Assuming an average wholesale price (AWP) less 20% plus $3.00, calculate the charges for the following items:

   a. 30 tabs; AWP $39.40/100 tabs _____

   b. 64 tabs; AWP $189.90/100 tabs _____

   c. 100 tabs; AWP $56.20/500 tabs _____

   d. 15 caps; AWP $94.20/30 caps _____

4. The following amounts are the actual costs of the products listed in the previous exercise. How much profit was made for each of the four products?

   a. $21.50/100 _____

   b. $73.25/100 _____

   c. $41.00/500 _____

   d. $67.20/30 _____

   e. What is the total profit? _____

5. What percentage profit is made on each of the following items?

   a. $20.00 cost and $24.00 charge _____

   b. $14.98 cost and $31.50 charge _____

   c. $1.24 cost and $8.99 charge _____

   d. $0.85 cost and $8.99 charge _____

6. How much profit is made for each of the following items?

   a. $64.50 cost and $84.20 charge _____

   b. $8.50 cost and $29.50 charge _____

   c. $1.20 cost and $8.62 charge _____

   d. $68.90 cost and $71.99 charge _____

   e. What is the total percentage profit for all four items? _____

7. Kelly's Pharmacy has an inventory of $139,400.00. Last week's sales totaled $41,200.00 and the profit was $6,123.00.

   a. What is Kelly's days' supply?

   _____

   b. If her inventory goal is 32 days, did she make it?

   _____

8. Greg's Pharmacy has an inventory of $183,245.00. His days' supply goal is 30. What do his weekly sales (in cost) need to be to make this goal?

   _____

9. What is the turnover rate if Greg's sales are $482,000.00 and his inventory average is $183,245.00?

   _____

10. A pharmacy has just opened on the corner of a busy intersection. It is projected that this pharmacy will have sales of $60,000.00 per week, and the cost of those sales will be $49,000.00 per week.

    a. If the days' supply goal is 34 days, how much inventory will the pharmacy be permitted to have on the shelves?

    _____

    b. If the cost of sales drops to $36,500.00, what will the pharmacy be permitted to have on the shelves?

    _____

WEB ACTIVITIES

1. Visit an online pharmacy such as RxUSA, at www.rxusa.com.

   a. What types of products can be purchased at such a site? _____

   _____

   _____

   b. Are prescriptions required? _____

   c. Is prescription benefit insurance accepted? _____

2. Visit the National Wholesale Drug Association (also called the Healthcare Distribution Management Association) Web site, at www.healthcaredistribution.org.

   a. What is this organization? _____

   _____

   b. On what types of news events does this organization report? _____

   _____

   c. Would this Web site be helpful to retail pharmacies or to hospital pharmacies? _____

   _____

3. Visit Express Scripts, at www.express-scripts.com.

   a. What is Express Scripts' mission statement? _____

   _____

   _____

   b. List three ways that the company makes prescription drugs more affordable. _____

   _____

   _____

4. Go to www.medicare.gov and find a provider for Part D Medicare drug prescription coverage in your region.

   a. What is the monthly premium? _____

   _____

   b. What is the annual deductible? _____

   _____

   c. Compare your findings with those of others in your class and summarize this comparison. _____

   _____

   _____

   _____

   d. Which program researched by your class would be best for your grandmother? _____

   _____

PUZZLING TERMINOLOGY

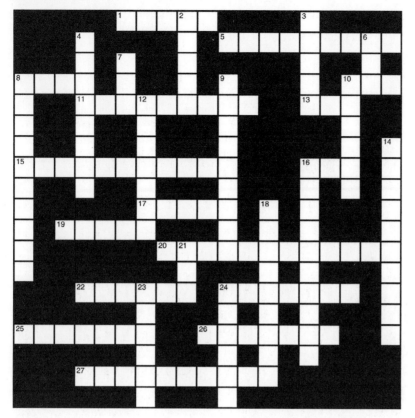

Down

2. device for connecting a computer to a remote computer via telephone lines

3. device used for getting information into the computer, such as a keyboard, mouse, or touch screen

4. reduced price

6. computer memory that is permanent and that contains essential operating instructions

7. average price that wholesalers charge the pharmacy for a drug

8. amount that insured must pay before the insurance company will consider paying its portion

9. claim form used for requesting the insurance company to provide coverage for a prescription

10. another word for gross profit

12. beginning inventory plus ending inventory, divided by two

14. merchant that supplies the pharmacy with numerous products from numerous manufacturers

16. monthly fee paid to the pharmacy by an insurer, to cover all of a patient's prescription costs

18. series of procedures for delivery of products

21. company that administers drug benefits from many different insurance companies

23. purchasing method in which drugs are ordered from the manufacturer

24. amount by which receipts exceed expenses

Across

1. vendor that agrees to make a specified percentage or dollar volume of purchases

5. entire stock of products on hand for sale at a given time

8. computer application that allows one to enter, retrieve, and query records

10. voluntary insurance program starting in January 2006 that provides partial coverage of prescriptions for patients eligible for Medicare

11. flat amount that the patient is to pay for each prescription

13. direct billing by the pharmacy to the customer's insurer

15. plan whereby the insured must pay a certain percentage of the prescription price

16. device used for manipulating computerized data input before output or storage

17. difference between the purchase price and the selling price

19. monetary worth

20. computer software programs that perform particular functions, such as word processing or spreadsheets

22. computer memory that holds information temporarily while it is being input and processed

24. device for creating hard copy or paper output

25. device for inputting images into the computer

26. display screen that provides a visual representation of data that have been input and/or processed

27. ordering of products for use or sale by the pharmacy

Extemporaneous Compounding

Chapter **8**

COMMUNICATION AND PHARMACY PRACTICE

1. Define the following terms:

   a. equilibrium _____

   b. parchment paper _____

   c. calibration _____

   d. topical _____

2. Research the properties of the following topical products, and determine what makes each different. Explain the difference in a memo to your classmates.

   a. Eucerin

   b. Aquaphor

   c. petrolatum

3. What is propylene glycol? Explain how it is used in topical preparations.

   _____

   _____

   _____

4. What is salicylic acid indicated for when it is added to topical preparations? What is in Whitfield's Ointment? _____

   _____

   _____

   _____

5. What effect will menthol have when added to topical preparations? How will it make the skin feel? _____

   _____

   _____

   _____

---

6. Phenol is used for two things when in a topical preparation. Research what it is used for at a low concentration and at a higher concentration.

_____

_____

_____

7. Research the ingredients in Magic Mouthwash (textbook Figure 8.1), and determine the action of each ingredient. (*Note:* The Magic Mouthwash formula given in the textbook is only one of several versions. Some compounds use Mylanta and/or lidocaine. You might find it interesting to call a compounding pharmacist in your area and compare his or her ingredients with those presented in the textbook.) _____

_____

_____

_____

WEB ACTIVITIES

1. Visit the Web site for the Professional Compounding Centers of America, at www.pccarx.com.

   a. What is the PCCA, and what services do its members provide? _____

   _____

   _____

   b. Find three interesting items in the device catalog to share with the class.

   _____

   _____

   c. List five applications for compounding medications._____

   _____

   _____

   d. Try to find at least one compounding pharmacy in your area, and jot down its name and contact information. In addition, explain how you found this information. _____

   _____

   _____

2. Visit the Web site for the *International Journal of Pharmaceutical Compounding,* at www.ijpc.com.

   a. Describe what is in the current issue of the journal._____

   _____

   _____

   b. View any past issue from the Free Sample Articles list, find an interesting article, and summarize the article.

3. Visit the Web site for the California Pharmacy and Compounding Center, at www.californiapharmacy.com.

    a. What is this site, and what is its specialty?_____

    _____

    _____

    b. What is a bio-identical hormone? _____

    _____

    _____

    c. Do bio-identical hormones require a prescription?_____

    _____

    d. What types of bio-identical hormones are compounded by this pharmacy?

    _____

    _____

IN THE LAB

Follow directions provided in the compounding recipes to accurately prepare mixtures of medicinal products in a pharmaceutically elegant form. This set of exercises provides an opportunity to experience the combining of various materials into medicinal products and product forms generally not available from a manufacturer.

Several recipes are provided that may be used in this exercise. For each compounding recipe, fill out a master formula sheet. Blank forms are found on pages 64–70.

Compounding equipment used in weighing, measuring liquids, grinding, and mixing, and so on, will be needed to complete these recipes. Students work in pairs to complete assigned compounds. Completed products will be checked by the instructor for technique, correctness of label, correct quantities of ingredients, and appearance.

1. Sugardyne

        Betadine Ointment 15 g
        Betadine Solution 6 mL
        sugar 60 g
        1. Measure all ingredients.
        2. Pool sugar (*Hint:* like potatoes and gravy).
        3. Mix ingredients from the middle of the pool outward. (*Remember:* neatness counts.)
        4. Place in 2 oz jar.
        5. Expires in 6 months.
        LABEL: Sugardyne
                      Date:
                      Exp:
                      "For topical use only"

2. salicyclic acid/Eucerin

> salicyclic acid 1 g
> hydrocortisone 1.2 g
> Eucerin 60 g
> 1. Measure ingredients.
> 2. Pool Eucerin cream (*Hint:* like potatoes and gravy).
> 3. Mix ingredients from the middle of the pool outward.
> 4. Place in 2 oz jar.
> 5. Expires in 6 months.
> LABEL: salicyclic acid/Eucerin
>   Date:
>   Exp:
>   "For topical use only"

3. simple syrup

> sucrose (i.e., granulated sugar) 850 g
> water in a sufficient quantity to make (QS ad) 1000 mL
> 1. Measure 500 mL tap water.
> 2. Place water in pan and bring to a boil.
> 3. Measure sucrose.
> 4. Add sucrose to boiling water.
> 5. Let pan cool slightly.
> 6. Pour into liter bottle. QS with water to total 1000 mL.
> 7. Expires in 6 months.
> LABEL: simple syrup, USP
>   Date:
>   Exp:
>   "Keep in refrigerator"

4. spironolactone oral suspension

> spironolactone 25 mg tablets
> #4 tablets
> simple syrup 50 mL
> water QS ad 100 mL
> 1. Crush tablets in mortar.
> 2. Measure simple syrup.
> 3. Add syrup into powdered spironolactone and mix well.
> 4. Add 25 mL water and mix well.
> 5. Pour into 4 oz bottle.
> 6. QS with water to total 100 mL.
> 7. Shake bottle well.
> 8. Expires in 30 days.
> LABEL: spironolactone oral suspension
>   conc. = 1 mg/mL
>   Date:
>   Exp:
>   "Shake well"

5. Modified Magic Mouthwash

> hydrocortisone powder 100 mg (may use pwd or inj)
> nystatin suspension 100,000 units/25 mL
> Benadryl Elixir QS ad 200 mL
> 1. Measure all ingredients.
> 2. Mix all ingredients in mortar.
> 3. Pour into 8 oz bottle.
> 4. Expires in 230 days.
> LABEL: Modified Magic Mouthwash
>   Date:
>   Exp:
>   "Shake well"

6. allopurinol oral suspension

> allopurinol 100 mg tablets
> #5 tablets
> simple syrup QS ad 100 mL
> 1. Crush tablets in mortar.
> 2. Add the simple syrup gradually and mix to uniform suspension.
> 3. Place in 4 oz bottle.
> 4. Expires in 14 days.
> LABEL: allopurinol oral suspension
>   conc. = 5 mg/mL
>   Date:
>   Exp:
>   "Shake well"
>   "Keep in refrigerator"

7. allergy cream

> menthol 60 mg
> triamcinolone cream 0.1% 60 g
> Cetaphil lotion QS 180 mL
> 1. Weigh menthol and crush in mortar.
> 2. Add 1–2 drops of alcohol to dissolve menthol.
> 3. Add approximately 1 oz of Cetaphil lotion.
> 4. Add half of triamcinolone cream and mix.
> 5. Mix other half of cream and some lotion, and pour into bottle.
> 6. QS to 180 mL with Cetaphil. Shake well as you add.
> 7. Expires in 6 months.
> LABEL: allergy cream
>   Date:
>   Exp:
>   "Shake well"
>   "For topical use only"

MASTER FORMULA SHEET

PRODUCT _____ MTC LOT NUMBER _____

_____
LABEL: Date MFG: _____

STRENGTH: _____
_____

QUANTITY MFG: _____
_____

	MANUFACTURER'S LOT NUMBER	INGREDIENTS	AMOUNT NEEDED	WEIGHED OR MEASURED BY	CHECKED BY
1					
2					
3					
4					
5					
6					
7					
8					

DIRECTIONS FOR MANUFACTURING

Manufactured by _____
Approved by _____
Date _____

_____
Auxiliary Labeling:
_____

MASTER FORMULA SHEET

PRODUCT _____ MTC LOT NUMBER _____

_____

LABEL: Date MFG: _____

STRENGTH: _____

QUANTITY MFG: _____

	MANUFACTURER'S LOT NUMBER	INGREDIENTS	AMOUNT NEEDED	WEIGHED OR MEASURED BY	CHECKED BY
1					
2					
3					
4					
5					
6					
7					
8					

DIRECTIONS FOR MANUFACTURING

Manufactured by _____
Approved by _____
Date _____

_____

Auxiliary Labeling:
_____

MASTER FORMULA SHEET

PRODUCT _____ MTC LOT NUMBER _____

_____

LABEL: Date MFG: _____

STRENGTH: _____

QUANTITY MFG: _____

	MANUFACTURER'S LOT NUMBER	INGREDIENTS	AMOUNT NEEDED	WEIGHED OR MEASURED BY	CHECKED BY
1					
2					
3					
4					
5					
6					
7					
8					

DIRECTIONS FOR MANUFACTURING

Manufactured by _____
Approved by _____
Date _____

_____

Auxiliary Labeling:
_____

MASTER FORMULA SHEET

PRODUCT _____ MTC LOT NUMBER _____

_____
LABEL: Date MFG: _____

                STRENGTH: _____
                          _____

                QUANTITY MFG: _____
                          _____

	MANUFACTURER'S LOT NUMBER	INGREDIENTS	AMOUNT NEEDED	WEIGHED OR MEASURED BY	CHECKED BY
1					
2					
3					
4					
5					
6					
7					
8					

DIRECTIONS FOR MANUFACTURING

Manufactured by _____
Approved by _____
Date _____

_____
Auxiliary Labeling: _____
_____

MASTER FORMULA SHEET

PRODUCT _____ MTC LOT NUMBER _____

LABEL: Date MFG: _____

STRENGTH: _____

QUANTITY MFG: _____

	MANUFACTURER'S LOT NUMBER	INGREDIENTS	AMOUNT NEEDED	WEIGHED OR MEASURED BY	CHECKED BY
1					
2					
3					
4					
5					
6					
7					
8					

DIRECTIONS FOR MANUFACTURING

Manufactured by _____
Approved by _____
Date _____

_____

Auxiliary Labeling:

_____

MASTER FORMULA SHEET

PRODUCT _____ MTC LOT NUMBER _____

_____

LABEL: Date MFG: _____

STRENGTH: _____

QUANTITY MFG: _____

	MANUFACTURER'S LOT NUMBER	INGREDIENTS	AMOUNT NEEDED	WEIGHED OR MEASURED BY	CHECKED BY
1					
2					
3					
4					
5					
6					
7					
8					

DIRECTIONS FOR MANUFACTURING

Manufactured by _____

Approved by _____

Date _____

_____

Auxiliary Labeling: _____

_____

MASTER FORMULA SHEET

PRODUCT _____ MTC LOT NUMBER _____

_____

LABEL: Date MFG: _____

                                     STRENGTH:

                                     _____

                                     QUANTITY MFG:

                                     _____

	MANUFACTURER'S LOT NUMBER	INGREDIENTS	AMOUNT NEEDED	WEIGHED OR MEASURED BY	CHECKED BY
1					
2					
3					
4					
5					
6					
7					
8					

DIRECTIONS FOR MANUFACTURING

Manufactured by _____
Approved by _____
Date _____

_____

Auxiliary Labeling:

_____

PUZZLING TERMINOLOGY

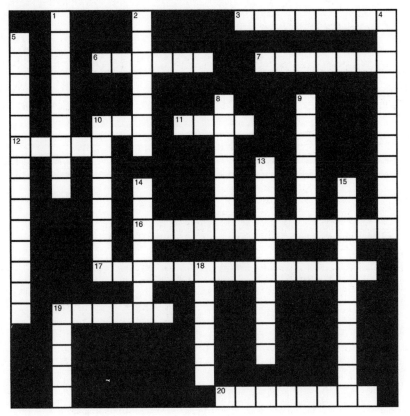

Down

1. dilution method in which drugs are combined using a mortar and pestle

2. instrument used to pick up small objects

4. process used to blend ingredients, often used in the preparation of creams and ointments

5. two-pan balance used for weighing material up to 5 kg, with a sensitivity rating of 100 mg

8. device used to weigh materials

9. ingredients to use and procedures to follow when compounding

10. flask used for measuring liquids

13. process reducing the particle size of a solid during the preparation of an ointment

14. long, thin, calibrated hollow tube used for measuring liquids having a volume of less than 1.5 mL

15. process of rubbing, grinding, or pulverizing a substance to create fine particles, generally by means of a mortar and pestle

18. club-shaped instrument used for mixing and grinding pharmaceutical ingredients

19. method for filling capsules in which the body of a capsule is repeatedly punched into a cake of medication until the capsule is full

Across

3. moon-shaped or concave appearance of a liquid in a graduate cylinder used in measurement

6. vessel used for mixing and grinding pharmaceutical ingredients

7. stainless steel, plastic, or hard rubber instrument used for transferring or mixing solid pharmaceutical ingredients

10. industry guidelines for ensuring that pharmacists prepare and dispense high-quality medications

11. flat, hard, nonabsorbent surface used for mixing compounds

12. variation above and below the target measurement

16. process of reducing the size of particles in a solid

17. compounding of medication in an appropriate quantity and dose form from several pharmaceutical ingredients

19. finely divided combination, or admixture, of drugs and/or chemicals ranging in size from extremely fine (No. 80) to very coarse (No. 8)

20. act of combining two substances

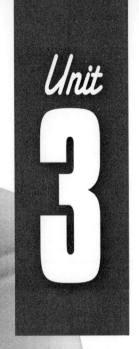

Unit 3

Institutional Pharmacy

Hospital Pharmacy Practice

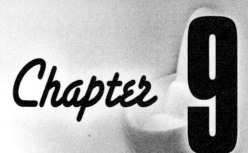

Chapter 9

WEB ACTIVITIES

1. Visit the American Society of Health-System Pharmacists Web site, at www.ashp.com. Describe the ASHP Advantage program. _____

   _____

   _____

   _____

2. Visit the Joint Commission on Accreditation of Healthcare Organizations Web site, at www.jcaho.com, and explore the information on hospital accreditation.

   a. What is accreditation for hospitals? _____

      _____

      _____

   b. What is the value of accreditation for hospitals? _____

      _____

      _____

      _____

      _____

   c. What seven accreditation decisions are made by the commission?

      _____

      _____

      _____

      _____

      _____

      _____

      _____

      _____

Medication Profile Review

To answer some of the following questions, you will need to use the appropriate drug reference materials. You might also find it helpful to refer to Appendix A, *Common Pharmacy Practice Abbreviations*.

1. Mr. Donald Wayne is an inpatient at Mt. Hope Hospital. Currently he is on these intravenous (IV) medications:

Order #	Medication	Route	Schedule	Date Started	Status
1	ciprofloxacin 400 mg	IV	q12h	1/19/XX	active
2	fluconazole 200 mg	IV	daily	1/19/XX	active
3	metronidazole 500 mg	IV	q8h	1/21/XX	active

   a. According to the patient's chart, the patient is receiving metronidazole.

      1) How many times a day is this drug given?_____

_____

      2) The patient receives an order for vancomycin 1 g daily. Is vancomycin compatible with metronidazole at the Y-site? Explain.

_____

_____

   b. Name a brand name for each of the drugs listed.

      1) ciprofloxacin _____

      2) fluconazole_____

      3) metronidazole _____

   c. Over how long should fluconazole be infused? _____

_____

   d. Are there oral dose forms for these IV medications?

      1) ciprofloxacin _____

      2) fluconazole_____

      3) metronidazole _____

Medication Orders

The exercises in this section provide you with an opportunity to practice extracting information from a medication order and entering information into a patient medication profile. If a computer is available, then the instructor may want each student to enter the orders into a computerized profiling system. However, with or without a computer system, write the required information on each of the profile forms provided. (As needed, refer to Table 9.1, Minibag Administration Protocol, on pages 123–124.) The medication orders and profile forms follow.

1.

(✓)	START HERE	DATE	TIME	PROFILED BY:	FILLED BY:	CHECKED BY:	PATIENT NAME AND I.D.
		12/15/XX	0130				James, Art 556789 Room 1049-1

D5/2NS w/ 20 mEq KCl/L at 125 cc/hr

Septra DS 1 po bid x 7 days

HCTZ 50 mg po qAM

Dilantin 100 mg IV tid

MOM 30 ml po prn constipation

Dr. Blood

Patient Profile

Patient Name:
Room Number:
ID:
Allergy:

Medication Ordered	Med/Soln	Type Soln	Fluid	Route	Frequency/Rate	Expiration of Soln	Duration	Comments

2.

(✓)	START HERE →	DATE 12/15/XX	TIME 0130	PROFILED BY:	FILLED BY:	CHECKED BY:	PATIENT NAME AND I.D. Taylor, Matt 689045 Room 609-1

morphine 8 mg IV q6-8h prn pain

Ancef 1 g IV q8h x 48 hr

D5LR + 10 mEq KCl/L at 75 cc/hr

Vasotec 2.5 mg IV q8h prn
systolic BP greater than 150
diastolic BP greater than 110

Tylenol ES po 1 q4h prn temp greater than 101°

Procardia 10 mg SL prn

Dr. Shoe

Patient Profile

Patient Name:
Room Number:
ID:
Allergy:

Medication Ordered	Med/ Soln	Type Soln	Fluid	Route	Frequency/ Rate	Expiration of Soln	Duration	Comments

3.

START HERE (✓)	DATE	TIME	PROFILED BY:	FILLED BY:	CHECKED BY:	PATIENT NAME AND I.D.

PATIENT NAME AND I.D.: Adams, Ashley
373744
Room 403-1

DATE 5/18/XX **TIME** 1600

D5NS + 40 g mag sulfate at 50 cc/hr
ampicillin 2 g IV q6h
Brethine 2.5 mg po q4h
Peri-Colace po 1 bid prn constipation
PNV (prenatal vitamins) po 1 daily
Vistaril 50 mg po q6h prn
Phenergan 25 mg PR q6h prn N/V

Dr. Grad

Patient Profile

Patient Name:
Room Number:
ID:
Allergy:

Medication Ordered	Med/ Soln	Type Soln	Fluid	Route	Frequency/ Rate	Expiration of Soln	Duration	Comments

Name _____

PATIENT NAME AND I.D.

Tyson, Margaret
373744
Room 620

START HERE (✓)	DATE 12/3/XX	TIME 0950	PROFILED BY:	FILLED BY:	CHECKED BY:

diagnosis acute GI bleed
allergies NKA
Zantac 150 mg in D5W 250 ml at 11 ml/hr
D5 1/2 NS w/ KCl 30 mEq/l at 100 ml/hr
Phenergan 25 mg IV q4–6h prn nausea
Demerol 50–75 mg q4h prn pain

Dr. S. Hammett

Patient Profile

Patient Name:
Room Number:
ID:
Allergy:

Medication Ordered	Med/ Soln	Type Soln	Fluid	Route	Frequency/ Rate	Expiration of Soln	Duration	Comments

5.

(✓)	START HERE ➔	DATE	TIME	PROFILED BY:	FILLED BY:	CHECKED BY:	PATIENT NAME AND I.D.
		12/3/XX	0915				Riggers, Jason 384743 Room 143

Procardia XL 60 mg po q AM
Xanax 0.25 mg po daily
Paxil 20 mg po daily
Colace 100 mg po qhs
PT three times a week
Ambien 5 mg po qhs

Dr. S. Hammett

Patient Profile

Patient Name:
Room Number:
ID:
Allergy:

Medication Ordered	Med/ Soln	Type Soln	Fluid	Route	Frequency/ Rate	Expiration of Soln	Duration	Comments

6.

PATIENT NAME AND I.D.	Cutt, Carrie 377344 Room 418				
	CHECKED BY:	FILLED BY:	PROFILED BY:	TIME	DATE
				1015	12/6/XX

Urocaps 3.0g q6h to start at noon
npo after midnight
bathroom privileges
change IV fluid to NS w/ KCl 10 mEq/L
Restoril 15 mg po tonight

Dr. S. Hammett

Patient Profile

Patient Name:
Room Number:
ID:
Allergy:

Medication Ordered	Med/ Soln	Type Soln	Fluid	Route	Frequency/ Rate	Expiration of Soln	Duration	Comments

Patient Profile

Patient Name:
Room Number:
ID:
Allergy:

Medication Ordered	Med/ Soln	Type Soln	Fluid	Route	Frequency/ Rate	Expiration of Soln	Duration	Comments

Medication Administration Record (MAR)

The medication administration record (MAR) documents the medications administered to patients. This document will list items such as the route of administration, time to start each medication, and time to stop each medication (if included in the order); the MAR is a duplicate copy of the medication order. This is part of the patient chart and is a legal document. These records are usually printed on a 24-hour basis and list the medications and administration times for 24 hours. Once a medication is administered, the nurse notes the time administered and initials the document. Scheduled drugs have listed times of administration, but *prn* (i.e., as needed) drugs do not have listed times. Table 9.2 (pages 124–125) lists the most frequent MAR administration times. This table provides standard times, unless the physician order states otherwise. Figure 9.1 (pages 85–86) is an example of a computerized MAR. Note that *q* generally means "around the clock" (e.g., q8h), whereas *tid* will mean "during waking hours."

This exercise will give you an opportunity to build a patient MAR by reading the included orders and placing the appropriate information in the MAR form. A blank form is provided for each of the patients in this exercise. The MAR forms follow the orders. If computers with pharmacy software are available, then the instructor may want the students to enter these orders into a computerized MAR.

FIGURE 9.1 Example of a Computerized MAR

MT. HOPE HOSPITAL

MEDICATION RECORD

IM		SQ	
A-Left Deltoid	E-Left Gluteus	J-Abdomen	M-LT Arm
B-Right Deltoid	F-Right Gluteus	K-RT Arm	N-LT Leg
C. Left Thigh	G-RT Ventrogluteal	L- RT Leg	
D- Right Thigh	I-LT Ventrogluteal		

NURSE VERIFICATION SIGNATURE:

03/15/XX 0800 to 03/16/XX 0759

START DATE & TIME TO STOP DATE & TIME	GENERIC NAME, STRENGTH, DOSAGE FORM / DOSE DIRECTIONS / TRADE NAME(S), COMMENTS		TBG / INITIAL	ROUTE FREQ.	1ST 0730-1530	2ND 1530-2330	3RD 2330-0730
03/03 0000 03/22 2359 #47	NS AMPICILLIN/SULBACTAM INFUSE OVER: 60MIN USE FOR UNASYN	50 ML 1.5 GM		IV Q6H PGY	12	18	00 06
03/08 0600 #62	DEXTROSE 5% METHYLDOPATE INFUSE OVER: 60MIN ALDOMET	100 ML 500 MG		IV Q6H PGY	12	18	00 06
03/03 0900 #49	FAMOTIDINE 40MG/5ML GIVE: 20 MG=2.5 ML PEPCID			NG Q12H	09	21	
03/03 1400 #50	PHENYTOIN 100MG/4ML GIVE: 100 MG=4 ML DILANTIN SUSP			NG Q8H	14	22	06
03/05 0800 #57	METOCLOPRAMIDE HCL 5MG/ML GIVE: 10 MG=2 ML REGLAN			IV Q6H	08 14	20	02
03/05 1400 #59	NIFEDIPINE 10MG GIVE: 10 MG=1 CAPSULE ADALAT/PROCARDIA USE FOR PROCARDIA			ORAL Q8H	14	22	06
03/10 2100 #71	DOCUSATE SODIUM 100MG/30ML GIVE: 100 MG=30 ML DSS/COLACE			ORAL BID	09	21	
02/25 0400 #5	ACETAMINOPHEN 325MG GIVE: 650 MG=2 TABLET TYLENOL PRN T > 101			ORAL Q4H PRN			
02/27 1900 #13	MAGNESIUM HYDROXIDE SUSP 30ML U/D GIVE: 30 ML LOC/MOM FOR CONSTIPATION MOM			ORAL DAILY PRN			
02/27 1900 #14	AL-MG OH &SIMETHICONE SUSP 30ML U/D GIVE: 30 ML MAALOX PLUS/MYLANTA			ORAL DAILY PRN			
02/28 1000 #23	ENALAPRILAT 1.25MG/ML GIVE: 1.25 MG=1 ML VASOTEC S&P > 150			IV Q6H PRN			

**ALLERGIES: NKA **

PT: HUDSON, LANDER
ACCOUNT # 32547698   RM: 275-2
MD: BLADDER, GALLE
NSI

DX: INT. RA CEREBRAL BLEEDING
PAGE 1   *CONTINUED*

(continues)

Name   Date   • *Chapter 9*   **85**

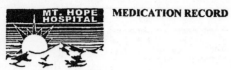

MT. HOPE HOSPITAL

MEDICATION RECORD

IM		SQ	
A-Left Deltoid	E-Left Gluteus	J-Abdomen	M-LT Arm
B-Right Deltoid	F-Right Gluteus	K-RT Arm	N-LT Leg
C. Left Thigh	G-RT Ventrogluteal	L- RT Leg	
D- Right Thigh	I-LT Ventrogluteal		

03/15/XX   0800   to   03/16/XX   0759

NURSE VERIFICATION SIGNATURE:

START DATE & TIME TO STOP DATE & TIME	GENERIC NAME, STRENGTH, DOSAGE FORM DOSE DIRECTIONS TRADE NAME(S), COMMENTS	TBG Δ/ INITIAL	ROUTE FREQ.	1ST 0730-1530	2ND 1530-2330	3RD 2330-0730
03/02 2100 #48	ARTIFICIAL TEARS OPTH SOL 15ML 8TL GIVE: *AS DIRECTED TEARS/LIQUIFILM		OPH DAILY PRN			
03/04 1000 #52	BISACODYL 10MG GIVE: 10 MG=1 SUPPOSITORY DULCOLAX		RTL PRN			
03/05 1100 #60	NIFEDIPINE 10MG GIVE: 10 MG=1 CAPSULE ADALAT/PROCARDIA PRN SBP) 150 *SL/NG**		ORAL Q2H PRN			
03/07 2334 #63	PROMETHAZINE HCL 25MG/ML GIVE: 12.5 MG=0.5 ML PHENERGAN MAY CAUSE DROWSINESS		IV Q2H PRN			
03/08 1600 #63	PROMETHAZINE HCL 25MG/ML GIVE: 25 MG=1 ML PHENERGAN MAY CAUSE DROWSINESS **MAY GIVE IV OR IM **		IM Q4H PRN			
03/09 1800 #67	LORAZEPAM 2MG/ML GIVE: 1-2 MG=0.5-1 ML ATIVAN PRN AGITATION, VENT DYSYNCHONY		IV Q4H PRN			

**ALLERGIES: NKA **
PT: HUDSON, LANDER
   ACCOUNT # 32547698   RM: 275-2
   MD: BLADDER, GALLE   DX: INT. RA CEREBRAL BLEEDING
   NSI   PAGE 2   *CONTINUED*

1.

START HERE	DATE 3/6/XX	TIME 0540	PROFILED BY:	FILLED BY:	CHECKED BY:	PATIENT NAME AND I.D.

(✓)	
	admit to 7E or 7W
	burns to hands, arms, face
	allergies: NKA
	whirlpool in AM
	Silvadene cream bid to wounds
	D5 1/2 NS w/ 20 KCl/L at 125 cc/hr
	Zantac 50 mg IV q8h
	morphine sulphate 2–4 mg IV q2h prn pain
	ampicillin 1 g IV q6h
	gentamicin 85 mg IV q8h

Patient: Reff, Mary 742153 Room 748-1

START HERE	DATE 3/6/XX	TIME 0540	PROFILED BY:	FILLED BY:	CHECKED BY:	PATIENT NAME AND I.D.

(✓)	
	Procardia 10 mg bite and swallow prn
	Sys greater than 150
	Dias greater than 110
	MVI 1 po daily
	zinc 200 mg po daily
	reg diet when taking po Percocet q4–6h prn
	Dr. P. Brown

Patient: Reff, Mary 742153 Room 748-1

2.

START HERE	DATE 4/6/XX	TIME 0730	PROFILED BY:	FILLED BY:	CHECKED BY:	PATIENT NAME AND I.D.

(✓)	
	Admit per Dr. Cook
	Dx MI
	Allergy Codeine
	Nitrol 2% 1/2" q6h off 0000 0600
	nitroglycerin 0.4 mg SL
	SBP greater than 170 DBP greater than 100
	Tylenol gr X po q6h po prn
	MOM 30 mL po prn
	1/2 NS w/ 20 mEq KCl/L at 50 mL/hr
	Dr. Cook

Patient: Johnson, Steve 268703 Room 328

3.

START HERE	DATE 4/5/XX	TIME 1000	PROFILED BY:	FILLED BY:	CHECKED BY:	PATIENT NAME AND I.D.

(✓)	
	admit
	Dx pneumonia
	Claforan 1 g IV q8h
	erythromycin 500 mg IV q6h
	D5 1/2 NS at 122 cc/hr
	Tylenol 650 mg po q4h prn pain or temp greater than 101

Patient: Spoker, Tom 104324 Room 232

START HERE →	DATE 4/5/XX	TIME 1000		PROFILED BY:	FILLED BY:	CHECKED BY:	PATIENT NAME AND I.D.
(✓)							

continue home meds
digoxin 0.125 mg po daily
hydralazine 75 mg po tid
Zantac 150 mg po bid
ASA 81 or 325 mg (choose one or the other) EC daily
Maalox 30 cc po q4h prn indigestion

G. Roger, MD

Spoken, Tom
1049324
Room 232

4.

START HERE →	DATE 4/6/XX	TIME 1300		PROFILED BY:	FILLED BY:	CHECKED BY:	PATIENT NAME AND I.D.
(✓)							

admit to Dr. Cook

Solu-Medrol 125 mg IVPB q8h x 4 doses
albumin 25 g IVPB followed w/ 40 mg Lasix
Biaxin 500 mg po q12h
Rocephin 1 g IVPB daily
albuterol aerosol q4h WA
D5½NS at 100 cc/hr x 4 then 60 cc/hr
Tylenol gr X po q4h T° greater than 101 or mild pain
Restoril 15 mg po qhs
Zantac 150 mg po bid 30 min ac + hs

Taylor, Mark
7642197
Room 649-1

START HERE →	DATE 4/6/XX	TIME 1300		PROFILED BY:	FILLED BY:	CHECKED BY:	PATIENT NAME AND I.D.
(✓)							

KCl 10 mEq 2 po qAM

J. Cook, MD

Taylor, Mark
7642197
Room 649-1

Medication Administration Record

Start date & time to stop date & time	Generic Name, Strength, Dose Form, Dose Directions, Trade Names, Comments	Route & Frequency	Day 0730–1530	Evening 1530–2330	Noc 2330–0730

Medication Administration Record

NAME:
ACCOUNT NO.:
RM NO.:

Allergy:

Start date & time to stop date & time	Generic Name, Strength, Dose Form, Dose Directions, Trade Names, Comments	Route & Frequency	Day 0730–1530	Evening 1530–2330	Noc 2330–0730

Medication Administration Record

Start date & time to stop date & time	Generic Name, Strength, Dose Form, Dose Directions, Trade Names, Comments	Route & Frequency	Day 0730–1530	Evening 1530–2330	Noc 2330–0730

Name _____   Date _____   • *Chapter 9*   **91**

Medication Administration Record

NAME:
ACCOUNT NO.:
RM NO.:

Allergy:

Start date & time to stop date & time	Generic Name, Strength, Dose Form, Dose Directions, Trade Names, Comments	Route & Frequency	Day 0730–1530	Evening 1530–2330	Noc 2330–0730

Medication Administration Record

Start date & time to stop date & time	Generic Name, Strength, Dose Form, Dose Directions, Trade Names, Comments	Route & Frequency	Day 0730–1530	Evening 1530–2330	Noc 2330–0730

Name   Date

Medication Distribution System

A unit dose is an ordered amount of medication in a dose that is in as ready-to-administer form as possible. Usually a 24-hour supply is delivered to or made available at patient care units.

These exercises will give you an opportunity to review orders to determine important pharmacy-related information, evaluate patient drawers for needs in filling a 24-hour supply, and practice filling patient drawers.

Unit Dose Orders

1. Use the following inpatient physician order to answer these questions:

(✓)	START HERE	DATE 10/16/XX	TIME 1500	PROFILED BY:	FILLED BY:	CHECKED BY:	PATIENT NAME AND I.D.
							Erwin, Tammy 0213-45 Room 300

Continue home meds:
(1) Capoten 12.5 mg po q12h
(2) nystatin cream to affected area tid
(3) digoxin 0.125 mg po daily
(4) nafcillin 1 g IV q6h
(5) enteric-coated aspirin gr X po daily

Smith, MD

    a. Identify the items of importance to the pharmacy by listing the corresponding numbers from the physician order.

    _____

    _____

    b. For each appropriate item, record the number of units needed for a 24-hour supply.

    _____

    _____

2. Use the following inpatient physician order to answer these questions:

(✓)	START → HERE	DATE 10/16/XX	TIME 1300		PROFILED BY:	FILLED BY:	CHECKED BY:	PATIENT NAME AND I.D.

Start following meds ASAP:
(1) hydralazine 10 mg IV q6h
(2) Emete-Con 50 mg IM q2–3h prn nausea
(3) D5½NS c̄ 20 mEq KCl at 50 mL/hr
(4) vital signs q shift
(5) npo after midnight

Blood, MD

Patient: Brooks, Thomas 00261-13 Room 502-2

a. Identify the items of importance to the pharmacy by listing the corresponding numbers from the physician order.

_____

_____

b. For each appropriate item, record the number of units needed for a 24-hour supply.

_____

_____

3. Use the following inpatient physician order to answer these questions:

(✓)	START → HERE	DATE 10/16/XX	TIME 1000		PROFILED BY:	FILLED BY:	CHECKED BY:	PATIENT NAME AND I.D.

(1) X-ray of kidneys
(2) fluids ad lib
(3) Pyridium 200 mg po tid
(4) urinalysis AM
(5) SMX-TMP 800 mg/160 mg po bid
(6) movement ad lib

Jones, MD

Patient: Wise, Kerry 00338-89 Room 504

a. Identify the items of importance to the pharmacy by listing the corresponding numbers from the physician order.

_____

_____

b. For each appropriate item, record the number of units needed for a 24-hour supply.

_____

_____

4. Use the following inpatient physician order to answer these questions:

(✓)	START HERE →	DATE 10/16/XX	TIME 1400	PROFILED BY:	FILLED BY:	CHECKED BY:	PATIENT NAME AND I.D.

Morris, Ronald
00334-83
Room 128-2

    (1) hydromorphone 2 mg q6h prn pain
    (2) Lasix 20 mg AM
    (3) keep L foot elevated
    (4) physical therapy AM
    (5) Zovirax ointment 5% apply to lesions q3h

                Smith, MD

a. Identify the items of importance to the pharmacy by listing the corresponding numbers from the physician order.

_____

_____

b. For each appropriate item, record the number of units needed for a 24-hour supply.

_____

_____

5. Use the following inpatient physician order to answer these questions:

(✓)	START HERE →	DATE 10/16/XX	TIME 1200	PROFILED BY:	FILLED BY:	CHECKED BY:	PATIENT NAME AND I.D.

Johnson, Tony
00325-77
Room 404-1

    (1) percussion twice daily
    (2) Ventolin Repetabs 4 mg q12h
    (3) acetaminophen 650 mg q4–6h prn
    (4) fluids ad lib
    (5) demonstrate use of Ventolin inhaler

                Hart, MD

a. Identify the items of importance to the pharmacy by listing the corresponding numbers from the physician order.

_____

_____

b. For each appropriate item, record the number of units needed for a 24-hour supply.

_____

_____

Cart Filling

This exercise will allow you to practice determining what is needed in the patient medication drawer. Complete the total daily quantity ordered and the amount to post for each item.

Drug	Amount Left in Drawer	Daily Quantity	Post/Add
1. ibuprofen 600 mg po q8h	2	_____	_____
2. Colace 100 mg liq po bid POS*	1	_____	_____
3. ferrous sulfate 325 mg po tid	0	_____	_____
4. doxycycline 100 mg po q12h	1	_____	_____
5. prednisone 7.5 mg po qAM	0	_____	_____
6. Benadryl 25 mg po qhs	1	_____	_____
7. Amoxil 250 mg po tid	0	_____	_____
8. Lasix 40 mg po qAM	1	_____	_____
9. Zantac 150 mg po bid	2	_____	_____
10. dexamethasone 2 mg IV q6h IVS	1	_____	_____
11. heparin flush IV q8h prn	0	_____	_____
12. Reglan 10 mg po ac & hs	2	_____	_____
13. Aldomet 250 mg po q8h	1	_____	_____
14. hydralazine 75 mg po q12h	0	_____	_____
15. Clinoril 200 mg po q12h	2	_____	_____
16. allopurinol 300 mg po qAM	0	_____	_____
17. captopril 6.25 mg po q8h prn	0	_____	_____
18. heparin flush IV q4h	3	_____	_____
19. Zantac 150 mg po bid	0	_____	_____
20. Reglan 10 mg po ac & hs	0	_____	_____
21. Theo-Dur 200 mg po bid	1	_____	_____
22. Vistaril 25 mg po q4h prn	3	_____	_____
23. Lopressor 25 mg po q8h POS*	0	_____	_____
24. DiaBeta 5 mg po qAM	0	_____	_____
25. Clinoril 200 mg po tid	1	_____	_____
26. Procardia 10 mg bite and swallow q4h prn	2	_____	_____
27. propranolol 10 mg po q8h	0	_____	_____
28. Keflex 500 mg po q6h	2	_____	_____
29. heparin 3000 units subcutaneous q12h POS*	0	_____	_____
30. Lopressor 25 mg po q12h POS*	0	_____	_____
31. Aldomet 125 mg liq po q8h	1	_____	_____
32. Pen-Vee K 500 mg po q6h	2	_____	_____

* oral special

Unit Dose Filling: Patient Fill List

In this activity, your instructor will partially fill some or all of the following patient drawers. You should finish filling the drawers with the appropriate quantities of medications and record the items added to each drawer. To prevent drug diversion, note any medications that are controlled drugs and should not be dispensed in the unit dose drug cart. Some drawers may be left empty to indicate a new patient.

1. Commons, Beth
    00276-28
    Room 420-1

Order	Daily Quantity	Post/Add
Benylin cough syrup q6h	4	_____
Cipro 750 mg q12h	2	_____
Dalmane 15 mg daily hs	1	_____
Norgesic Forte daily in the AM	1	_____
Filled by: _____		

2. Reese, Michael
    00335-79
    Room 211-2

Order	Daily Quantity	Post/Add
Reglan syrup 10 mg tid ac	3	_____
Motrin 800 mg q6h	4	_____
Dalmane 30 mg daily hs	1	_____
MOM 30 mL qhs prn	1	_____
allopurinol 200 mg daily in the AM	1	_____
Filled by: _____		

3. Love, Tanya
    00333-90
    Room 361-1

Order	Daily Quantity	Post/Add
Lasix 40 mg daily in the AM	1	_____
Clinoril 150 mg bid	2	_____
Valium 2 mg daily hs	1	_____
Keflex 500 mg q6h	4	_____
Filled by: _____		

4. Stallone, Stacy
    00336-88
    Room 117

Order	Daily Quantity	Post/Add
Toprol 100 mg q12h	2	_____
acetaminophen 325 mg q6h	4	_____
Dimetapp tablet po q12h	1	_____
Diuril 500 mg po bid	2	_____
Filled by: _____		

5. Roof, William
    00335-88
    Room 112-1

Order	Daily Quantity	Post/Add
Aventyl 10 mg daily in the AM	1	_____
ascorbic acid 250 mg daily	1	_____
Mycelex-7 Troch qid	1	_____
guaifenesin syrup 200 mg q4h	6	_____
Filled by: _____		

6. Cutt, Carrie
   00283-35
   Room 272

Order	Daily Quantity	Post/Add
Pen-Vee K 500 mg qid	4	_____
Motrin 400 mg q6h	4	_____
Zyloprim 100 mg bid	2	_____
multivitamin daily	1	_____
Filled by: _____		

For this next set of orders, fill in the daily quantity needed for each medication per the orders given. Your instructor will partially fill some or all of these patient drawers. Finish filling the drawers with the appropriate quantities of medications, and record the items added to each drawer.

7. Cato, Inez
   00270-22
   Room 206-1

Order	Daily Quantity	Post/Add
doxycycline caps 100 mg po q12h	_____	_____
multivitamins daily	_____	_____
ibuprofen 400 mg q8h	_____	_____
Dulcolax 5 mg suppository daily hs	_____	_____
DiaBeta 1.25 mg daily in the AM	_____	_____
Filled by: _____		

8. Jeffery, George
   00320-72
   Room 501-2

Order	Daily Quantity	Post/Add
Procardia 30 mg XL daily	_____	_____
Dyazide daily	_____	_____
Naldecon Tabs q12h 1 now	_____	_____
Dalmane 15 mg daily hs	_____	_____
Filled by: _____		

9. Rish, Randy
   00335-82
   Room 550

Order	Daily Quantity	Post/Add
Cipro 250 mg bid	_____	_____
Voltaren 50 mg tid	_____	_____
Mylanta 60 mL ac & hs	_____	_____
Reglan 10 mg 30 min AC	_____	_____
Filled by: _____		

10. Erwin, Tammy
    00293-45
    Room 300

Order	Daily Quantity	Post/Add
Coumadin 2 mg daily in the AM	_____	_____
MS Contin 30 mg q12h	_____	_____
diltiazem 60 mg tid	_____	_____
glycerin suppository prn	_____	_____
Filled by: _____		

11. Murphy, Peggy
00334-84
Room 321-2

Order	Daily Quantity	Post/Add
Zantac 300 mg bid	_____	_____
Cytotec 100 mg q6h	_____	_____
Feldene 40 mg q12h	_____	_____
Dalmane 15 mg hs prn	_____	_____
Filled by: _____		

12. Hine, Herman
00311-63
Room 380

Order	Daily Quantity	Post/Add
Benadryl 25 mg qhs	_____	_____
Allopurinol 300 mg qAM	_____	_____
Vistaril 25 mg q4h	_____	_____
propranolol 10 mg q8h	_____	_____
Lotrimin 1% cream tid	_____	_____
Filled by: _____		

Repackaging Medications

Oral Specials

This is an exercise in repackaging drug products for oral dosing. References for repackaging guidelines are provided by the American Society of Health-System Pharmacists (ASHP) in the *ASHP Technical Assistance Bulletin on Single Unit and Unit Dose Packages of Drugs*.

This exercise includes completing a unit dose repackaging control log (page 104) for the 10 drugs listed for preparation. You will record all 10 drugs on the log as if a 3-day supply were to be prepared. In addition, prepare the doses and labels and include all auxiliary labels that apply. Prepare your work for inspection. Consider these points when determining expirations:

- All liquids have a 30-day expiration unless otherwise stated.
- All tablets have a 90-day expiration unless otherwise stated.
- Syringes kept at room temperature have a 30-day expiration (anything up to and including 10 mL).
- Reconstituted antibiotics have a 5-day expiration in syringes and go into the refrigerator.
- Reconstituted bottles of antibiotics have a 14-day expiration. Read the label.
- Oral specials over 10 mL go into bottles and have a 90-day expiration at room temperature.

The lot number will list PO, the last number in the year, the month, the day, and the number of the drug prepared (e.g., 01 for the first of the day, 02 for the second, 03 for the third). *Example:* for October 10, 2007, and the second drug prepared, the lot number will be PO7101002. The following example (Figure 9.2) is done for you as a guide:

FIGURE 9.2 Repacking Control Log Example

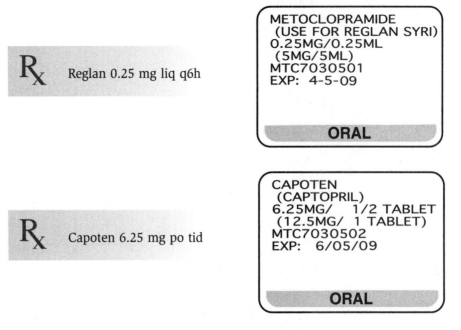

R_x   Reglan 0.25 mg liq q6h

METOCLOPRAMIDE
  (USE FOR REGLAN SYRI)
0.25MG/0.25ML
  (5MG/5ML)
MTC7030501
EXP: 4-5-09

ORAL

R_x   Capoten 6.25 mg po tid

CAPOTEN
  (CAPTOPRIL)
6.25MG/   1/2 TABLET
  (12.5MG/ 1 TABLET)
MTC7030502
EXP: 6/05/09

ORAL

REPACKAGING CONTROL LOG
DEPARTMENT OF PHARMACEUTICAL SERVICES

PHARMACY LOT NUMBER	DRUG-STRENGTH DOSE FORM	MANUFACTURER AND LOT NUMBER	EXP. DATE MANUF. MTC	RESULTING CONC.	QUANTITY	PREP. BY CK'D
MTC P07040501	metoclopramide oral soln	Roxane 194 ABI	3/10 / 4/4/09	0.25 mg / 0.25 mL (5 mg / 5 mL)	12	aVT
MTC P07060502	captopril 12.5 mg tabs	Squibb 12 RAV8	7/11 / 6/5/09	6.25 mg / 1/2 tab (12.5 mg / 1 tab)	9	aVT

Name   Date   • *Chapter 9*   **101**

1. ℞ Nystatin 500,000 units/5 mL tid

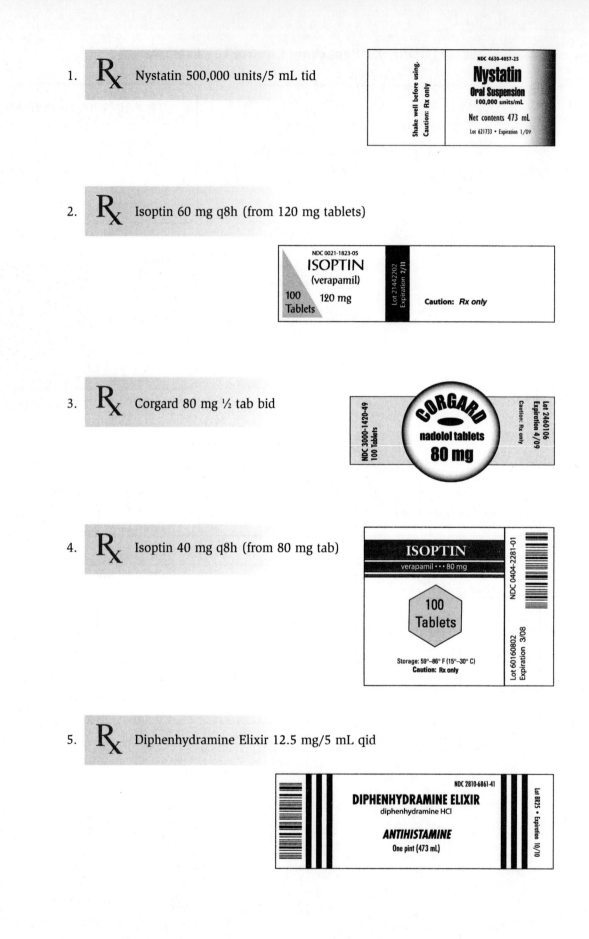

NDC 4630-4057-25
Nystatin
Oral Suspension
100,000 units/mL
Net contents 473 mL
Lot 621733 • Expiration 1/09

Shake well before using.
Caution: Rx only

2. ℞ Isoptin 60 mg q8h (from 120 mg tablets)

NDC 0021-1823-05
ISOPTIN
(verapamil)
100 Tablets   120 mg
Lot 21442202
Expiration 2/11
Caution: *Rx only*

3. ℞ Corgard 80 mg ½ tab bid

NDC 3000-1420-49
100 Tablets
CORGARD
nadolol tablets
80 mg
Caution: Rx only
Lot 2460106
Expiration 4/09

4. ℞ Isoptin 40 mg q8h (from 80 mg tab)

ISOPTIN
verapamil • • • 80 mg
100 Tablets
NDC 0404-2281-01
Lot 60160802
Expiration 3/08
Storage: 59°–86° F (15°–30° C)
Caution: Rx only

5. ℞ Diphenhydramine Elixir 12.5 mg/5 mL qid

NDC 2810-6861-41
DIPHENHYDRAMINE ELIXIR
diphenhydramine HCl
ANTIHISTAMINE
One pint (473 mL)
Lot 8R25 • Expiration 10/10

6. ℞ potassium chloride solution 40 mEq bid

POTASSIUM CHLORIDE SOLUTION
Sugar Free

Each 15 mL supplies 40 mEq each of potassium
and chloride as potassium chloride.
ONE PINT

Lot 0093
Expiration 11/10
NDC 3100-3113-43

Caution: Rx only

7. ℞ Lanoxin Elixir 25 mcg daily

NDC 1900-1460-80
LANOXIN
ELIXIR
(digoxin)
60 mL
Each mL contains 50 mcg (0.05 mg).
Lot 62L71
Expiration 10/09

8. ℞ Septra liquid 160 mg q6h

NDC 0008-1021-06
SEPTRA
Oral Suspension
(sulfamethoxazole–trimethoprim)
Each 5 mL contains sulfamethoxazole
200 mg and trimethoprim 40 mg.
Lot 41109096
Expiration 10/08
Cherry Flavor   437 mL

9. ℞ Norgesic Forte 1 q6h

NDC 0089-0233-50
NORGESIC FORTE
100 Tablets
Each tablet contains
orphenadrine citrate
50 mg, aspirin 770 mg,
caffeine 60 mg.
Lot 38273 • Expiration 10/10

10. ℞ DiaBeta 2.5 mg bid (from 5 mg tab)

DIAΒETA
(glyburide)
5 mg
500 Tablets
Caution: Rx only
NDC 009-0502-05
Control: 790052
Expiration 10/11

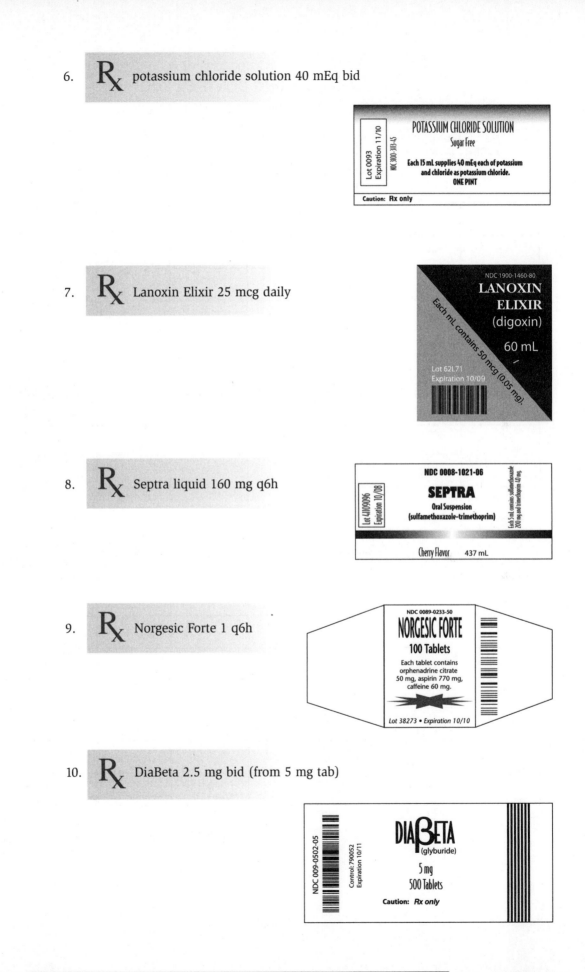

REPACKAGING CONTROL LOG
DEPARTMENT OF PHARMACEUTICAL SERVICES

PHARMACY LOT NUMBER	DRUG-STRENGTH DOSE FORM	MANUFACTURER AND LOT NUMBER	EXP. DATE MANUF. MTC	RESULTING CONC.	QUANTITY	PREP. BY CK'D

IV Specials

The IV special (IVS) is a single dose in a labeled syringe prepared under sterile conditions, that is, under laminar airflow hood conditions. The syringe is given an overfill volume of 0.1 mL to account for drug volume lost in the needle and syringe hub when the needle is attached and the drug administered. The overfill is not indicated on the prepackaging control log.

Expiration dates will depend on the agent being prepared. Information concerning reconstitutions can be found in Table 9.3 (pages 125–126). Expiration dates can be obtained from Table 9.1 (pages 123–124). Table 9.4 (page 127) provides guidelines for preparing IV specials. (Read the extreme right column of Table 9.1, headed IVS, to determine if the drug can be prepared as an IV special.) Table 9.4 outlines specific expiration dates. The time used for preparing IV specials is 1600. This corresponds to the present chart exchange time. Therefore all IV specials will have the appropriate expiration date and the time of expiration of 1600. This only affects IV specials, not dilutions made by the pharmacy. The determined expiration date is reduced by 1 day (24 hours). The prepared syringe is generally maintained in the patient tray and not refrigerated. If the drug is unused and returned to the pharmacy, then it is destroyed even if it has not expired; it is not recycled to another patient.

Generally a 3-day supply is prepared. However, the procedure may vary from institution to institution.

Some drugs cannot be refrigerated and therefore will not be made as an IVS for storage under refrigeration.

The IVS label will contain the following information:
- stock bottle name
- generic or trade name as ordered
- amount ordered
- concentration of stock bottle
- lot number (start with IV)
- expiration date and time
- auxiliary labels/notes (e.g., must dilute further)

The lot number will list IV, the last number in the year, the month, the day, and the number of the drug prepared (e.g., 01 for the first of the day, 02 for the second, 03 for the third). *Example:* for March 7, 2007, and the fifth drug prepared, the lot number will be IV7030705.

When preparing the drug, use the smallest syringe possible. Remember, each IVS will contain 0.1 mL overfill.
- If the total volume including overfill is less than or equal to 1 mL, use a tuberculin (TB) (1 mL) syringe.
- If the total volume including overfill is greater than 1 mL but less than or equal to 3 mL, then use a 3 mL syringe.
- If the total volume including overfill is greater than 3 mL but less than or equal to 5 mL, then use a 5 mL syringe.
- If the total volume including overfill is greater than 5 mL but less than or equal to 10 mL, then use a 10 mL syringe.

Standardized dosing will decrease errors and decrease the number of doses to be made. For example, when calculating the standard dose for pediatric patients using a dexamethasone injection (0.5 mg/mL), assume a 0.45–0.55 mg dose range. The standard dose is 0.5 mg, and the volume is 0.1 mL.

1. Using the repackaging control log on page 107, log the eight repackaged medications listed below. You will need to calculate some of the medications to arrive at a final concentration. Log each medication for a 3-day supply. The following is an example:

```
LANOXIN INJECTION
 (DIGOXIN)
 0.125MG/0.5ML
  (0.25MG/ML)
 I8031601
 EXP 4/16/09    1600
```

REPACKAGING CONTROL LOG
DEPARTMENT OF PHARMACEUTICAL SERVICES

PHARMACY LOT NUMBER	DRUG-STRENGTH DOSE FORM	MANUFACTURER AND LOT NUMBER	EXP. DATE MANUF. MTC	RESULTING CONC.	QUANTITY	PREP. BY CK'D
IV7041601	(Digoxin) Lanoxin 250mcg/mL	BW A49381	9/10 4/16/09	0.25 mg/mL) 0.125 mg/0.5mL	3	DCB

a. gentamicin 5 mg IV q12h (dilute for IV use); use a concentration of 20 mg/2 mL

b. vancomycin 20 mg IV q24h; use a concentration of 50 mg/mL

c. tobramycin 48 mg IV q8h; use a concentration of 40 mg/mL

d. heparin 3000 units subcutaneous q12h; use a concentration of 5000 units/mL

e. dexamethasone 0.8 mg IV q12h; use a concentration of 4 mg/mL

f. penicillin G 50,000 units IV q12h; use a concentration of 250,000 units/mL

g. Claforan 200 mg IV q8h; use a concentration of 200 mg/mL

h. phenobarbital 9 mg IV q24h; use a concentration of 65 mg/mL

REPACKAGING CONTROL LOG
DEPARTMENT OF PHARMACEUTICAL SERVICES

PHARMACY LOT NUMBER	DRUG-STRENGTH DOSE FORM	MANUFACTURER AND LOT NUMBER	EXP. DATE MANUF. MTC	RESULTING CONC.	QUANTITY	PREP. BY / CK'D

2. Your instructor will select three of the medications in the last exercise to be prepared as IVS syringes. Prepare only 1 unit of each and cap with a syringe cap. Write a label for each and attach it to the prepared syringe. Make an additional copy of the labels to use as a study copy.

Labels   Syringe Labels

Mt. Hope Pharmacy Services

Patient: _____ ID. No._____ Rm. No. _____

Prepared: _____ Date:_____

Expiration: _____   By:

Mt. Hope Pharmacy Services

Patient: _____ ID. No._____ Rm. No. _____

Prepared: _____ Date:_____

Expiration: _____   By:

Mt. Hope Pharmacy Services

Patient: _____ ID. No._____ Rm. No. _____

Prepared: _____ Date:_____

Expiration: _____   By:

3. Write labels with the following information for (a) gentamicin, (b) heparin, and (c) phenobarbital. Use the order information from exercise 1 (page 106).

- drug injection
- concentration of dose ordered and original concentration used
- lot number
- expiration date and time

a. gentamicin

Mt. Hope Pharmacy Services
Patient: _____ ID. No. _____ Rm. No. _____
Prepared: _____ Date: _____
Expiration: _____   By:

b. heparin

Mt. Hope Pharmacy Services
Patient: _____ ID. No. _____ Rm. No. _____
Prepared: _____ Date: _____
Expiration: _____   By:

c. phenobarbital

```
┌──────────────────────────────────────────────────────┐       ┌──────────────────────────────┐
│              Mt. Hope Pharmacy Services               │       │                              │
│                                                        │       │                              │
│  Patient: _____  ID. No._____  Rm. No. ____ │    │                              │
│                                                        │       │                              │
│  Prepared: _____    Date:_____            │       │                              │
│                                                        │       │                              │
│                                                        │       │                              │
│                                                        │       └──────────────────────────────┘
│                                                        │
│                                                        │
│                                                        │
│                                                        │
│  Expiration:                        By:                │
└──────────────────────────────────────────────────────┘
```

Pediatric and Neonatal Dosing

Calculate the drug dose for the following pediatric patients. These exercises are very important, because math errors can result in an adverse reaction or death in the hospital. Review the tables and examples in Chapter 5 or abbreviations in Appendix A if necessary to solve the problems.

1. How many grams are in 1 lb?

    _____

2. J. B. is a 3-year-old weighing 37 lb. What is his weight in kg?

    _____

3. A. K. is a 21-day-old neonate weighing 2.6 lb.

    a. The physician order reads ampicillin 100 mg/kg/dose IV q6h. How much ampicillin should be sent up per dose for this baby?

        _____

    b. The physician orders gentamicin 5 mg/kg/day IV q12h. How much gentamicin should be sent up per dose?

        _____

4. T. N. is a 14-month-old girl weighing 25 lb. The recommended dose of ceftriaxone is 50 mg/kg/day IV given once a day. What would her dose be?

    _____

5. S. R. is a 3-year-old weighing 35 lb. The physician order indicates amoxicillin po 50 mg/kg/day tid. Amoxicillin comes as a 125 mg/5 mL suspension. How much amoxicillin would be dispensed in an oral syringe for one dose? (Indicate milligrams per dose and milliliters per dose.)

    _____

6. B. B. is a 53-day-old neonate weighing 2.5 kg.

    a. The physician orders aminophylline 6 mg/kg IV loading dose, then 2 mg/kg IV q8h. How many milligrams would you prepare for each dose?

    _____

    b. Then the physician orders morphine 0.37 mg IV 12–24 hr prn pain. How many mg/kg/dose is this?

    _____

7. T. B. is a 15-year-old boy brought in because of seizures. He weighs 120 lb. The physician wants to load him with phenobarbital at 15 mg/kg and then 12 hours later start 3 mg/kg/day on a bid schedule. What is his loading and daily maintenance dose?

    _____

8. D. A. is a 1-day-old neonate weighing 800 g. The physician orders cefotaxime 150 mg/kg/day IV q8h. How many mg/kg/dose should be prepared?

    _____

9. Q. P. is a 10-year-old girl admitted for asthma. She weighs 90 lb. The physician orders methylprednisolone (Solu-Medrol) 2 mg/kg/day IV q6h.

    a. What is her total daily dose?

    _____

    b. How many milligrams are in one dose?

    _____

10. E. M. is an 8-year-old girl weighing 63 lb. The physician orders amoxicillin 40 mg/kg/day po tid. The amoxicillin you will use is a 250 mg/5 mL suspension.

    a. How many milligrams will one dose be?

    _____

    b. How many milliliters will one dose be?

    _____

Adult Total Parenteral Nutrition (TPN)

For the following two patients, calculate volumes of each component that will constitute the adult total parenteral nutrition (TPN). It is suggested that students work independently on calculations, but be assigned to groups for preparation of the product. Each student in a group should have a part in measuring components and injecting them into the fluid admixture. Use the supply information provided in Figure 9.5 (pages 115–116) and Table 9.5 (page 127) as needed.

1. Queen's TPN (Figure 9.3, page 112) will be formulated using peripheral formulation for peripheral administration. Dextrose 40% will be used to formulate a 6% solution with a total volume of 1100 mL. Use 50 mL of 10% lipids. Determine the number of milliliters for each of the ingredients on the TPN sheet (Figure 9.3). Calculations will be checked by your instructor and technique observed during compounding.

    a. amino acids 25 g = _____ mL

    b. dextrose 40% = _____ mL

c. fat 10% = _____ mL

d. trace elements = _____ mL

e. multivitamins = _____ mL

f. sodium chloride = _____ mL

g. magnesium sulfate = _____ mL

h. potassium chloride = _____ mL

i. human insulin = _____ mL >

FIGURE 9.3 TPN Order for Queen

Adult Parenteral Nutrition Order Form
Mt. Hope Hospital
My Town, SC

Patient: *Queen, Dixie*
Room: *306-B*

Date: _____ Time: *1530*

☐ Consult Nutritional Support Service (Beeper 0349)

☐ Conduct Indirect Calorimetry Test

Central Formula (per liter)		Peripheral Formula (per liter)	
Amino Acids	40 g	Amino Acids	25 g
Dextrose	17.5% (600 kcals) *40%*	Dextrose	6% (200 kcals)
Fat 20%	125 mL (250 kcals)	Fat 20% *10%*	~~200 mL (400 kcals)~~ *50mL*
Standard Electrolytes*		~~Standard Electrolytes*~~ *See below*	
Trace Elements—4: 1 mL/day		Trace Elements—4: 1 mL/day	
Multivitamins—12: 10 mL/day		Multivitamins—12 10 mL/day	
		Osmolarity: 740 mOsm/L	
Total Volume _____ mL/day		Total Volume *1100* mL/day	

*Standard Electrolytes (per liter) Na: 50 mEq, Ca: 7.5 mEq, Cl: 45 mEq, Acetate: 45 mEq, Phos: 9 mM

Special Formulation (Indicate Total Daily Requirements)	Guidelines	General Rule
1. Amino Acids _____ g/day	0.5–2.5 g/kg/day	1 g/kg/day
Type _____		
2. Total Nonprotein		
Calories _____ kcals/day*	10–40 kcals/kg/day	25 kcals/kg/day
Dextrose _____ %	0–100%	65%
Fat _____ %	0–65%	35%
100%		100%
3. Total Volume _____ mL/day	Minimum Volume: 1 kcal/1.0 mL	

*Substrate must equal 100%.

Special Formulation—Electrolytes (check one)

☐ Standard Electrolytes/Liter

☐ Standard Electrolytes plus Additional Electrolytes

☐ Standard Electrolytes/Liter—No Potassium   ☑ Custom Electrolytes

Sodium Acetate	_____ mEq/day	Potassium Acetate	_____ mEq/day
Sodium Chloride	*10* mEq/day	Potassium Chloride	*20* mEq/day
Sodium Phosphate	_____ mEq/day	Potassium Phosphate	_____ mEq/day
Magnesium Sulfate	*8* mEq/day	Calcium Gluconate	_____ mEq/day

Multivitamins—12: (10 mL) per _____   Other _____
Trace Elements—4: (1 mL) per _____   Other _____

HUMAN REGULAR INSULIN *30* units/day

Phytonadione (Vit. K) 10 mg ☒ per *week*

OTHER _____

Special Instructions _____
Dr. Smith Jones

M.D.   Pharmacy Must Receive TPN Orders by 12 Noon
76016153

2. Itchy's TPN (Figure 9.4, page 114) will be a special formulation using 8.5% amino acids, dextrose prepared to 20%, and 20% lipids. The lipids will not be mixed as was the case in the 3-in-1 fluids, but in this instance the original bottle will be sent to the floor. Total volume will be 1000 mL. Determine the number of milliliters for each of the ingredients on the TPN sheet (Figure 9.4). Calculations will be checked by the instructor and technique observed during compounding.

a. amino acids 30 g = _____ mL

b. dextrose 40% = _____ mL

c. sterile water = _____ mL

d. sodium chloride = _____ mL

e. magnesium sulfate = _____ mL

f. potassium chloride = _____ mL

g. calcium gluconate = _____ mL

h. trace elements = _____ mL

Adult Parenteral Nutrition Order Form
Mt. Hope Hospital
My Town, SC

Patient: *Itchy, Johnny*
Room: *457-a*

Date: _____ Time: _1045_

☐ Consult Nutritional Support Service (Beeper 0349)

☐ Conduct Indirect Calorimetry Test

Central Formula (per liter)		Peripheral Formula (per liter)	
Amino Acids	40 g	Amino Acids	25 g
Dextrose	17.5% (600 kcals)	Dextrose	6% (200 kcals)
Fat 20%	125 mL (250 kcals)	Fat 20%	200 mL (400 kcals)
Standard Electrolytes*		Standard Electrolytes*	
Trace Elements—4: 1 mL/day		Trace Elements—4: 1 mL/day	
Multivitamins—12: 10 mL/day		Multivitamins—12: 10 mL/day	
		Osmolarity: 740 mOsm/L	
Total Volume _____ mL/day		Total Volume _____ mL/day	

*Standard Electrolytes (per liter) Na: 50 mEq, Ca: 7.5 mEq, Cl: 45 mEq, Acetate: 45 mEq, Phos: 9 mM

Special Formulation (Indicate Total Daily Requirements) | **Guidelines** | **General Rule**
1. Amino Acids _30_ g/day | 0.5–2.5 g/kg/day | 1 g/kg/day
   Type *8.5 Travasol*

2. Total Nonprotein
   Calories _____ kcals/day* | 10–40 kcals/kg/day | 25 kcals/kg/day

   Dextrose _20_ % | 0–100% | 65%
   Fat _20_ % | 0–65% | 35%
   100% | | 100%

3. Total Volume _1000_ mL/day | Minimum Volume: 1 kcals/1.0 mL
*Substrate must equal 100%.

Special Formulation—Electrolytes (check one)

☐ Standard Electrolytes/Liter   ☐ Standard Electrolytes plus
                                          Additional Electrolytes

☐ Standard Electrolytes/Liter—No Potassium   ☑ Custom Electrolytes

Sodium Acetate	____ mEq/day	Potassium Acetate	____ mEq/day
Sodium Chloride	_20_ mEq/day	Potassium Chloride	_40_ mEq/day
Sodium Phosphate	____ mEq/day	Potassium Phosphate	____ mEq/day
Magnesium Sulfate	_4_ mEq/day	Calcium Gluconate	_10_ mEq/day

Multivitamins—12: (10 mL) per _____   Other _____
Trace Elements—4: (1 mL) per *Day*   Other _____

HUMAN REGULAR INSULIN _____ units/day

Phytonadione (Vit. K) 10 mg IM per _____

OTHER _____

Special Instructions _____
    Dr. Smith Jones
M.D.   Pharmacy Must Receive TPN Orders by 12 Noon
76016153

FIGURE 9.5 Adult TPN Order Form

Adult Parenteral Nutrition Order Form
Mt. Hope Hospital
My Town, SC

Patient: _____
Room: _____

Date: _____ Time: _____

☐ Consult Nutritional Support Service (Beeper 0349)

☐ Conduct Indirect Calorimetry Test

Central Formula (per liter)
   Amino Acids   40 g
   Dextrose   17.5% (600 kcals)
   Fat 20%   125 mL (250 kcals)
   Standard Electrolytes*
   Trace Elements—4: 1 mL/day
   Multivitamins—12: 10 mL/day

   Total Volume _____ mL/day

Peripheral Formula (per liter)
   Amino Acids   25 g
   Dextrose   6% (200 kcals)
   Fat 20%   200 mL (400 kcals)
   Standard Electrolytes*
   Trace Elements—4: 1 mL/day
   Multivitamins—12: 10 mL/day
   Osmolarity: 740 mOsm/L
   Total Volume _____ mL/day

*Standard Electrolytes (per liter) Na: 50 mEq, Ca: 7.5 mEq, Cl: 45 mEq, Acetate: 45 mEq, Phos: 9 mM

Special Formulation (Indicate Total Daily Requirements)

	Guidelines	General Rule
1. Amino Acids _____ g/day	0.5–2.5 g/kg/day	1 g/kg/day
Type _____		
2. Total Nonprotein		
Calories _____ kcals/day*	10–40 kcals/kg/day	25 kcals/kg/day
Dextrose _____%	0–100%	65%
Fat _____%	0–65%	<u>35%</u>
100%		100%
3. Total Volume _____ mL/day	Minimum Volume: 1 kcals/1.0 mL	

*Substrate must equal 100%.

Special Formulation—Electrolytes (check one)

☐ Standard Electrolytes/Liter

☐ Standard Electrolytes/Liter—No Potassium

☐ Standard Electrolytes plus
   Additional Electrolytes

☐ Custom Electrolytes

Sodium Acetate	_____ mEq/day	Potassium Acetate	_____ mEq/day
Sodium Chloride	_____ mEq/day	Potassium Chloride	_____ mEq/day
Sodium Phosphate	_____ mEq/day	Potassium Phosphate	_____ mEq/day
Magnesium Sulfate	_____ mEq/day	Calcium Gluconate	_____ mEq/day

Multivitamins—12: (10 mL) per _____
Trace Elements—4: (1 mL) per _____

Other _____
Other _____

HUMAN REGULAR INSULIN _____ units/day

Phytonadione (Vit. K) 10 mg IM per _____

OTHER _____

Special Instructions _____
_____

M.D.
76016153

Pharmacy Must Receive TPN Orders by 12 Noon

(continues)

FIGURE 9.5 (*CONTINUED*)

M.V.I-12 10 mL* contains: (indicates adult RDA)

1.	Ascorbic Acid	100.0 mg	(45 mg)
2.	Vitamin A	3300.0 units	(4000–5000 units)
3.	Vitamin D	200.0 units	(4000–5000 units)
4.	Thiamine	3.0 mg	(1.0–1.5 mg)
5.	Riboflavin	3.6 mg	(1.1–1.8 mg)
6.	Pyridoxine	4.0 mg	(1.6–2.0 mg)
7.	Niacin	40.0 mg	(12–20 mg)
8.	Pantothenic Acid	15.0 mg	(5–10 mg)
9.	Vitamin E	10.0 units	(12–15 units)
10.	Biotin	60.0 mg	(150–300 mcg)
11.	Folic Acid	400.0 mcg	(400 mcg)
12.	Vitamin B_{12}	5.0 mcg	(3 mcg)

*Provides 100% of AMA guidelines for parenteral vitamin supplementation.

Trace Elements 1 mL contains: (AMA daily recommendations)

1. Zinc 5.0 mg (2.5–4 mg)   3. Manganese 0.5 mg (0.15–0.8 mg)
2. Copper 1.0 mg (0.5–1.5 mg)   4. Chromium 10.0 mcg (10–15 mcg)

INSTRUCTIONS FOR USING ORDER FORM

1. Check N S S CONSULT or INDIRECT CALORIMETRY (Metabolic Cart) if desired.

2. Order STANDARD CENTRAL or STANDARD PERIPHERAL FORMULAS by total **milliliters** per day. Nutritional components listed on form as per liter. Standard formulas include MVI, TE, and standard electrolytes.

3. Use SPECIAL FORMULATION section for any orders other than standard formulas including addition of electrolytes and other than standard electrolytes.

4. AMINO ACIDS ordered in **milliliters** per day. If a change in rate is desired, **then** place a new order for acid products (i.e., renal, hepatic, or HBC).

5. TOTAL NONPROTEIN CALORIES ordered as kcals per day. Specify percentage of total calories to be supplied by dextrose and percentage to come from lipids.

6. TOTAL VOLUME ordered in **milliliters** per day. If a change in rate is desired, **then** a new order form needs to be filled out to ensure the change is acknowledged by the IV pharmacy.

7. If either STANDARD ELECTROLYTES or STANDARD ELECTROLYTES — NO POTASSIUM are desired, check the appropriate box.

8. If CUSTOM ELECTROLYTES are desired, check the box and order total mEq per day. If STANDARD ELECTROLYTES PLUS ADDITIONAL ELECTROLYTES are desired, **then** check the appropriate box and specify additional electrolytes in mEq/day.

   Use standard electrolytes (per liter) listed under standard formulas as a guide. Note: 4.0 mEq of Na phosphate or 4.4 mEq K phosphate provides 3 mM phosphate.

9. MULTIVITAMINS and TRACE ELEMENTS should be ordered per day.

10. Specify INSULIN (in units/day) and VITAMIN K if desired; then outline any SPECIAL INSTRUCTIONS if applicable.

ALL TPN ORDERS RECEIVED IN THE PHARMACY BY 1200 WILL BE HUNG BETWEEN 1800 AND 2200 THE SAME DAY.

Pharmacy Use

Pediatric and Neonatal Nutritional Calculations and Preparations

In these exercises you will calculate ingredient levels for pediatric and neonatal parenteral feeding. Your instructor may assign a pediatric TPN (total parenteral nutrition) to be compounded or design one for student preparation. Use the supply information provided in Table 9.6, Neonatal Pharmacy Nutrition Supply List, on page 127, as a reference to make calculations for materials used in preparing a TPN.

Pediatric Nutrition Practice

1. An order was received for baby Brown, weighing 1264 g, and you are to prepare the lipids at 2 g/kg for 20 hours. The rate is 8.3 mL/hr.

    a. What volume of lipids would be drawn up in a syringe if 20% lipids are used?

    _____

    b. Calculate the following equivalencies to three significant figures, or three digits (i.e., 101, 10.1, 1.01, 0.101), for each answer:

    1) TrophAmine 6% amino acids 1.6 g = _____ mL

    2) dextrose 10% 4 g = _____ mL

    3) sodium chloride 8 mEq = _____ mL

    4) potassium phosphate 4.4 mEq = _____ mL

    5) potassium chloride 2 mEq = _____ mL

    6) magnesium sulfate 1 mEq = _____ mL

    7) calcium gluconate 2 mEq = _____ mL

    8) pediatric multivitamins 6.5 mL = _____ mL

    9) pediatric trace elements 0.1 mL = _____ mL

    10) heparin 0.5 units/mL = _____ mL

    c. Add all volumes together.

    _____

    d. Determine the volume of sterile water to be added by subtracting the total of the components volume from the total actual volume (TAV), 200 mL.

    _____

2. How many grams of amino acids are there if you have 250 mL of a 6% amino acid solution?

    _____

3. How many grams of dextrose are there in a 500 mL 10% solution?

    _____

4. What volume is needed for each of the following:

   a. NaCl 154 mEq _____

   b. potassium phosphate 20 mEq _____

   c. magnesium sulfate 10 mEq _____

5. A bag of TPN has 500 mL left in it at 1100 today; the rate is 75 mL/hr. When is the next bag due?

   a. day _____

   b. time _____

6. How long will a 250 mL bag last if the rate is 15 mL/hr?

   _____

7. How many grams of dextrose are there if you have 500 mL of a 70% dextrose solution?

   _____

Neonatal Nutrition Practice

1. How many grams of dextrose are there in 250 mL of a 10% solution?

   _____

2. How many grams of protein are there in 500 mL of a 6% TrophAmine solution?

   _____

3. If a TPN order calls for 12.5% dextrose, how many milliliters of the stock 50% dextrose will you need to fill this order if the total actual volume (TAV) is to be 275 mL?

   _____

4. How many grams of fat are in 200 mL of a 20% solution?

   _____

5. Baby Green is a 26-week gestation neonate weighing 700 g and is 3 days old. He is being treated for prematurity and respiratory distress syndrome, and sepsis cannot be ruled out. He is in critical condition and on a ventilator. A neonatologist has ordered hyperalimentation for him beginning today. Review the order (Figure 9.6, page 119), and calculate the caloric content ordered in kilocalories per day.

   a. dextrose 3.4 kcal/g = _____ kcal/day

   b. lipid 9 kcal/g = _____ kcal/day

   c. protein 4 kcal/g = _____ kcal/day

   d. total = _____ kcal/day

FIGURE 9.6 Fluid Order for Baby Green

MT. HOPE HOSPITAL
SPECIAL FLUID ORDER SHEET

DATE: _Nov. 10_   NICU   TIME: _____

PATIENT NO:_____   WEIGHT (KILOGRAMS): _0.7_

PATIENT NAME: _Baby Green_   AGE (DAYS): _____

COMPONENT	AMOUNT/KG/24 HR	LABEL	TOTAL ML
AMINO ACIDS ___TrophAmine___	0.5	0.35 g	_____
DEXTROSE (%) _50%_	_____	10%	_____
SODIUM CHLORIDE	1 mEq	0.7 mEq	_____
POTASSIUM PHOSPHATE	1.4 mEq	0.98 mEq	_____
POTASSIUM CHLORIDE	0.5 mEq	0.35 mEq	_____
MAGNESIUM SULFATE	0.25 mEq	0.175 mEq	_____
CALCIUM GLUCONATE	1 mEq	0.7 mEq	_____
PEDIATRIC MULTIVITAMINS	_____		6.5
TRACE ELEMENTS	_____		0.07
HEPARIN (BEEF)	1 unit/mL	75 units	_____
		TAV (TOTAL ACTUAL VOLUME)	_____
		TOTAL COMPONENTS	_____
STERILE WATER			_____
			_____

Fluid Infusion rate (mL/hr): _3_   **IV LIPIDS**

Volume of Fluids (TAV in mL): _75_   Lipids (g/kg/24 hr): _0.5_

Osmolarity: _____   Percent Lipid: _20%_ _____

Location of Line: (Peripheral) (Central)   Volume Lipid: _____

Infusion (hours): _20_

Dr. _____Smith_____

---

6. Review the neonatal hyperalimentation or TPN order for baby Green. Using the Neonatal Pharmacy Nutrition Supply List (Table 9.6, page 127), calculate the amount in milliliters of each ingredient to add.

   a. TrophAmine 6% = _____ mL

   b. dextrose 10% = _____ mL

   c. sodium chloride = _____ mL

   d. potassium phosphate = _____ mL

   e. potassium chloride = _____ mL

   f. potassium acetate = _____ mL

   g. magnesium sulfate = _____ mL

   h. calcium gluconate = _____ mL

   i. pediatric multivitamin injection = _____ mL

   j. neonatal trace elements = _____ mL

   k. heparin (beef) = _____ mL

   l. sterile water = _____ mL

   m. lipids 20% = _____ mL

7. Baby Taylor is a 30-week gestational neonate weighing 1500 g. She is 7 days old and is being treated for prematurity and pneumonia. She is on a ventilator and has a central percutaneous catheter (i.e., central line). Review the ordered TPN order (Figure 9.7), and calculate the caloric content ordered in kilocalories per day.

   a. dextrose 3.4 kcal/g = _____ kcal/day

   b. lipid 9 kcal/g = _____ kcal/day

   c. protein 4 kcal/g = _____ kcal/day

   d. total caloric content ordered = _____ kcal/day

FIGURE 9.7 Fluid Order for Baby Taylor

MT. HOPE HOSPITAL
SPECIAL FLUID ORDER SHEET

DATE: *June 11*   NICU   TIME: _____

PATIENT NO:_____   WEIGHT (KILOGRAMS): _1.5_____

PATIENT NAME: *Taylor Girl*_____   AGE (DAYS):_____

COMPONENT		AMOUNT/KG/24 HR	LABEL	TOTAL ML
AMINO ACIDS	*TrophAmine*	2.5	3.75g	
DEXTROSE (%) *50%*			17%	
SODIUM CHLORIDE		4 mEq	6 mEq	
POTASSIUM PHOSPHATE		2 mEq	3 mEq	
POTASSIUM CHLORIDE		2 mEq	3 mEq	
MAGNESIUM SULFATE		1 mEq	1.5 mEq	
CALCIUM GLUCONATE		1.75 mEq	2.63 mEq	
PEDIATRIC MULTIVITAMINS				6.5
TRACE ELEMENTS				0.15
HEPARIN (BEEF)				
			TAV (TOTAL ACTUAL VOLUME)	
			TOTAL COMPONENTS	
STERILE WATER				

Fluid Infusion rate (mL/hr): _8.9_   IV LIPIDS

Volume of Fluids (TAV in mL): _214_   Lipids (g/kg/24 hr): _1.5_

Osmolarity: _____   Percent Lipid: _20%_ _____

Location of Line: (Peripheral) (Central)   Volume Lipid: _____

Infusion (hours): _20_

Dr. _Smith_____

8. For baby Taylor, calculate the amount of milliliters of ingredients ordered, using the Neonatal Pharmacy Nutrition Supply List (Table 9.6, page 127).

   a. TrophAmine 6% = _____ mL

   b. dextrose 17% = _____ mL

   c. sodium chloride = _____ mL

   d. potassium phosphate = _____ mL

   e. potassium chloride = _____ mL

   f. potassium acetate = _____ mL

   g. magnesium sulfate = _____ mL

    h. calcium gluconate = _____ mL

    i. pediatric multivitamin injection = _____ mL

    j. neonatal trace elements = _____ mL

    k. heparin (beef) = _____ mL

    l. sterile water = _____ mL

    m. lipids 20% = _____ mL

9. Review the TPN order for Baby X (Figure 9.8, page 122). Calculate the amount in milliliters of ingredients ordered.

    a. TrophAmine 6% = _____ mL

    b. dextrose 12.5% = _____ mL

    c. sodium chloride = _____ mL

    d. potassium phosphate = _____ mL

    e. potassium chloride = _____ mL

    f. potassium acetate = _____ mL

    g. magnesium sulfate = _____ mL

    h. calcium gluconate = _____ mL

    i. pediatric multivitamin injection = _____ mL

    j. neonatal trace elements = _____ mL

    k. heparin (beef) = _____ mL

    l. sterile water = _____ mL

    m. lipids 20% = _____ mL

FIGURE 9.8 Fluid Order for Baby X

MT. HOPE HOSPITAL
SPECIAL FLUID ORDER SHEET

DATE: *June 11*   NICU   TIME: _____

PATIENT NO: _____   WEIGHT (KILOGRAMS): *1*

PATIENT NAME: *Baby X* _____   AGE (DAYS): _____

COMPONENT	AMOUNT/KG/24 HR	LABEL	TOTAL ML
AMINO ACIDS ___*TrophAmine*___	2.5	2.5 g	_____
DEXTROSE (%) *50%*		12.5%	_____
SODIUM CHLORIDE	6 mEq	6 mEq	_____
POTASSIUM PHOSPHATE	2.8 mEq	2.8 mEq	_____
POTASSIUM CHLORIDE	2 mEq	2 mEq	_____
MAGNESIUM SULFATE	3 mEq	3 mEq	_____
CALCIUM GLUCONATE	3.2 mEq	3.2 mEq	_____
PEDIATRIC MULTIVITAMINS	_____	_____	6.5
TRACE ELEMENTS	_____	_____	0.1
HEPARIN (BEEF)	_____		_____
		TAV (TOTAL ACTUAL VOLUME)	_____
		TOTAL COMPONENTS	_____
STERILE WATER			_____

Fluid Infusion rate (mL/hr): ___33___   **IV LIPIDS**

Volume of Fluids (TAV in mL): ___80___   Lipids (g/kg/24 hr): ___0___

Osmolarity: _____   Percent Lipid: _____ _____

Location of Line: (Peripheral) (Central)   Volume Lipid: _____

Infusion (hours): ___24___

Dr. ___*Smith*___

10. Calculate the amount in milliliters of ingredients ordered in this neonatal TPN:

     a. amino acids 10% 9 g = _____ mL

     b. dextrose 12.5% 20% = _____ mL

     c. sodium chloride 23 mEq = _____ mL

     d. potassium phosphate 4.4 mEq = _____ mL

     e. potassium chloride 2 mEq = _____ mL

     f. magnesium sulfate 2 mEq = _____ mL

     g. calcium gluconate 0.5 mEq = _____ mL

     h. pediatric multivitamins 5 mL = _____ mL

     i. pediatric trace elements 0.15 mL = _____ mL

     j. heparin 1 unit/mL = _____ mL

     k. the amount of sterile water to be added, given TAV = 480 mL and a rate of 20 mL/hr: _____ mL

TABLE 9.1 Minibag Administration Protocol

Agent	Volume	Infusion Rate	EXP	IVS (IV Special)
acyclovir (Zovirax)**	≤ 1 g; 50 mL	60 min	24 hr RT	no
amikacin	≤ 500 mg; 100 mL	60 min	24 hr RT	no
	> 500 mg; 250 mL			
aminocaproic acid (Amicar)	≤ 2 g; 50 mL	30 min	24 hr RT	no
	> 2 g; 100 mL	30 min		
	> 5 g; 250 mL	30 min		
aminophylline bolus	≤ 250 mg; 50 mL	30 min	24 hr RT	no
	> 250 mg; 100 mL	30–60 min		
ampicillin*	≤ 1.5 g; 50 mL NS	60 min	8 hr RT	no
	> 1.5 g; 100 mL NS	60 min	72 hr REF	
ampicillin-sulbactam* (Unasyn)	≤ 1.5 g; 50 mL NS	60 min	8 hr RT	no
	> 1.5 g; 100 mL	60 min	72 hr REF	
aztreonam (Azactam)	≤ 1 g; 50 mL	60 min	48 hr RT	no
	> 1 g; 100 mL	60 min	7 day REF	
cefamandole (Mandol)	≤ 2 g; 50 mL	60 min	24 hr RT	no
	> 2 g; 100 mL	60 min	96 hr REF	
cefazolin (Ancef, Kefzol)	≤ 2 g; 50 mL	60 min	24 hr RT	yes
	> 2 g; 100 mL	60 min	96 hr RT	
cefonicid (Monocid)	≤ 2 g; 50 mL	30 min	24 hr RT	no
	> 2 g; 100 mL	30 min	72 hr REF	
cefoperazone (Cefobid)	≤ 3 g; 50 mL	30 min	24 hr RT	no
	> 3 g; 100 mL	30 min	120 hr REF	
cefotaxime (Claforan)	≤ 2 g; 50 mL	30 min	24 hr RT	yes
	> 2 g; 100 mL	30 min	120 hr REF	
ceftazidime (Fortaz, Tazidime)	≤ 2 g; 50 mL	60 min	24 hr RT	no
	> 2 g; 100 mL		7 day REF	
cefotetan (Cefotan)	≤ 1 g; 50 mL	60 min	24 hr RT	no
	> 1 g; 100 mL	60 min	96 hr REF	
ceftizoxime (Cefizox)	≤ 2 g; 50 mL	30 min	24 hr RT	no
	> 2 g; 100 mL	30 min	48 hr REF	
ceftriaxone (Rocephin)	≤ 2 g; 50 mL	30 min	72 hr RT	no
	> 2 g; 100 mL	30 min	10 day REF	
cefoxitin (Mefoxin)	≤ 2 g; 50 mL	30 min	24 hr RT	no
	> 2 g; 100 mL	30 min	48 hr REF	
cefuroxime (Zinacef)	≤ 750 mg; 50 mL	60 min	24 hr RT	no
	> 750 mg; 100 mL	60 min	48 hr REF	
cephalothin	≤ 2 g; 50 mL	30 min	24 hr RT	yes
	> 2 g; 100 mL	30 min	96 hr REF	
chloramphenicol (Chloromycetin)	≤ 2 g; 50 mL	30 min	24 hr RT	yes
	> 2 g; 100 mL	30 min	30 day REF	
cimetidine (Tagamet)	≤ 300 mg; 50 mL	30 min	48 hr RT	no
	> 300 mg; 100 mL	30 min	7 day REF	
clindamycin (Cleocin)	≤ 300 mg; 50 mL	30 min	16 day RT	no
	> 300 mg; 100 mL	30 min	30 day REF	
doxycycline (Vibramycin)	≤ 200 mg; 200 mL	60 min	24 hr RT	no
	> 200 mg; 250 mL	1.5 hr	72 hr REF	
erythromycin*	≤ 1 g; 100 mL NS	60 min	8 hr RT	no
lactobionate	> 1 g; 250 mL NS	1.5 hr		
famotidine (Pepcid)	≤ 40 mg; 100 mL	30 min	96 hr RT	yes
furosemide (Lasix)***	Do not exceed 4 mg/min		24 hr RT	no
gentamicin (Garamycin)	≤ 120 mg; 50 mL	30 min	96 hr RT	yes
	> 120 mg; 100 mL	30 min	30 day REF	
imipenem-cilastin (Primaxin)*	≤ 500 mg; 100 mL NS	60 min	10 hr RT	no
	> 500 mg; 250 mL NS	60 min	48 hr REF	

(continues)

*Denotes normal saline use only.
**Do not refrigerate.
***Protect from light.

Note: Prepare each agent in D$_5$W unless advised otherwise. RT indicates room temperature and REF indicates refrigeration.

Name _____ Date _____

TABLE 9.1 *(CONTINUED)*

Agent	Volume	Infusion Rate	EXP	IVS (IV Special)
methicillin (Staphcillin)	≤ 1 g; 50 mL	60 min	8 hr RT	yes
	> 1 g; 100 mL	60 min	96 hr REF	
methlydopa (Aldomet)	≤ 500 mg; 100 mL	60 min	24 hr RT	yes
	> 500 mg; 250 mL	24 hr		
metronidazole (Flagyl)**	500 mg RTU	60 min	Manuf.	no
	any other dose	60 min	24 hr RT	
mezlocillin	≤ 2 g; 50 mL	30 min	48 hr RT	no
	> 2 g; 100 mL	30 min	7 day REF	
nafcillin	≤ 1 g; 50 mL	60 min	24 hr RT	no
	> 1 g; 100 mL	60 min	96 hr REF	
oxacillin*	≤ 2 g; 50 mL NS	60 min	96 hr RT	no
	> 2 g; 100 mL NS	60 min	7 day REF	
penicillin	≤ 3 million units; 50 mL	30 min	24 hr RT	yes
IVS pentamidine (Pentam)	≤ 300 mg; 100 mL	60 min	24 hr RT	no
	> 300 mg; 250 mL	60 min		
piperacillin (Pipracil)	≤ 4 g; 50 mL	30 min	24 hr RT	no
	> 4 g; 100 mL	30 min	7 day REF	
potassium chloride	> 40 mEq; 100 mL	60 min	24 hr RT	no
ranitidine (Zantac)	≤ 50 mg; 50 mL	30 min	48 hr RT	no
	> 50 mg; 100 mL	30 min	10 day REF	
ticarcillin (Ticar)	≤ 3 g; 50 mL	60 min	24 hr RT	no
	> 3 g; 100 mL	60 min	72 hr REF	
ticarcillin-clavulanate potassium (Timentin)	≤ 3.1 g; 50 mL	60 min	24 hr RT	no
	> 3.1 g; 100 mL	60 min	72 hr REF	
tobramycin (Nebcin)	≤ 120 mg; 50 mL	30 min	24 hr RT	no
	> 120 mg; 100 mL	30 min	96 hr REF	
trimethoprim-sulfamethozaxole (Septra) **	Each 5 mL amp in each 75 mL	60–90 min	2 hr RT	no
	Each 5 mL amp in each 125 mL	60–90 min	6 hr RT	
vancomycin (Vancocin)	≤ 250 mg; 50 mL	60 min	96 hr RT	yes
	> 250 mg; 100 mL	60 min		
	> 1 g; 250 mL	60 min		

*Denotes normal saline use only.
**Do not refrigerate.

TABLE 9.2 Most Frequent MAR Administration Times

Common Hospital Codes	Administration Times
daily, qAM	0900
every other day, q48	0900 on day to be given
q3d, q4d, q5d, q6d	every 3rd, 4th, 5th, or 6th day
qw	every week
q4w	every 4 weeks (or once a month)
mxw	multiple days of the week
Coumadin dosed daily	1800
daily 6p	1800
qPM	1900
qhs	2100, or bedtime
bid	0900, 2100
tid	0900, 1300, 1700
qid	0900, 1300, 1700, 2100
q4	0100, 0500, 0900, 1300, 1700, 2100
5xd	0600, 1000, 1400, 1800, 2200
q6A	0600, 1200, 1800, 0000
q6B	0500, 1100, 1700, 2300
q6C	0200, 0800, 1400, 2000
q8A	0600, 1400, 2200

(continues)

TABLE 9.2 *(CONTINUED)*

Common Hospital Codes	Administration Times
q8B	0100, 0900, 1700
q12A	0900, 2100
q12B	0600, 1800
q12C	0500, 1700
q12D	1100, 2300
q12E	0200, 1400
qAMI	insulin dosed 30 minutes before breakfast
qPMI	insulin dosed 30 minutes before supper
WM1	with meals once a day, daily with a meal
WM2	with meals twice a day, bid with meals
WM3	with meals three times a day, tid with meals

TABLE 9.3 Reconstitutions

Medications	Vial	Add (mL)	to Make
ampicillin	10 g	44.5	1 g/5 mL
	2 g	9	1 g/5 mL
	1 g	4.5	1 g/5 mL
	500 mg	2.5	1 g/5 mL
ampicillin-sulbactam (Unasyn)	3 g	6.4	3 g/8 mL
	1.5 g	3.2	1.5 g/4 mL
aztreonam (Azactam)	2 g	7.4	1 g/5 mL
	1 g	3.8	1 g/5 mL
	500 mg	2.5	1 g/5 mL
cefamandole (Mandol)	2 g	9	1 g/5 mL
	1 g	4.5	1 g/5 mL
cefazolin (Ancef)	10 g	45.5	1 g/5 mL
	1 g	4.5	1 g/5 mL
	500 mg	2.5	1 g/5 mL
cefonicid (Monocid)	1 g	4.5	1 g/5 mL
cefoperazone (Cefobid)	2 g	9	1 g/5 mL
	1 g	4.5	1 g/5 mL
cefotaxime (Claforan)	10 g	47	1 g/5 mL
	1 g	4.5	1 g/5 mL
cefoxitin (Mefoxin)	10 g	45.5	1 g/5 mL
	2 g	9	1 g/5 mL
	1 g	4.5	1 g/5 mL
ceftazidime (Fortaz, Tazidime)	2 g	8.7	1 g/5 mL
	1 g	4.4	1 g/5 mL
	vent before and after		
ceftizoxime (Cefizox)	2 g	9	1 g/5 mL
	1 g	4.5	1 g/5 mL
ceftriaxone (Rocephin)	2 g	9	1 g/5 mL
	1 g	4.5	1 g/5 mL
	500 mg	2.5	1 g/5 mL

(continues)

TABLE 9.3 **Reconstitutions** (*CONTINUED*)

Medications	Vial	Add (mL)	to Make
cefuroxime (Zinacef)	1.5 g	16	90 mg/mL
	750 mg	8	90 mg/mL
cephalothin	20 g	108	1 g/6 mL
	2 g	11.2	1 g/6 mL
	1 g	5.6	1 g/6 mL
chloramphenicol	1 g	4.7	1 g/5 mL
doxycycline (Vibramycin)	200 mg	9.2	100 mg/5 mL
	100 mg	4.6	100 mg/5 mL
methicillin	4 g	5.7	1 g/2 mL
	1 g	1.5	1 g/2 mL
mezlocillin (Mezlin)	4 g	18.5	1 g/5 mL
	1 g	1.5	1 g/5 mL
nafcillin	10 g	44.5	1 g/5 mL
	2 g	9	1 g/5 mL
	1 g	4.5	1 g/5 mL
	500 mg	2.5	1 g/5 mL
pediatric multivitamins	50 mL	49	
	10 mL	9.4	
	vent		
penicillin G	note side of vial		
pentamidine	300 mg	5	300 mg/5 mL
piperacillin	4 g	18	1 g/5 mL
	3 g	13.5	1 g/5 mL
ticarcillin (Ticar)	20 g	47	1 g/3 mL
	3 g	7	1 g/3 mL
	1 g	2.5	1 g/3 mL
vancomycin	5 g	100	50 mg/mL

TABLE 9.4 Guidelines for Preparing Intravenous Specials (IVSs)

Medication	Concentration	Expiration Date
aminophylline dilution	10 mg/mL 3 mL TAV	1 day
cefazolin (Ancef, Kefzol)	200 mg/mL	4 days minus 1 day
cefotaxime (Claforan)	200 mg/mL	5 days minus 1 day
cephalothin	166.66 mg/mL	4 days minus 1day
cimetidine (Tagamet) minibag	6 mg/mL minibag	7 days
chloramphenicol injection	100 mg/mL	1 month minus 1 day
dexamethasone (Decadron)	4 mg/mL	1 month minus 1 day
dexamethasone dilution	0.5 mg/mL dilution	7 days
digoxin	100 mcg/mL (pediatric) 250 mcg/mL (adult)	1 month minus 1 day
digoxin dilution	20 mcg/mL dilution	7 days
gentamicin	10 mg/mL (pediatric) 40 mg/mL (adult)	20 days minus 1 day
heparin	10,000 units/mL	1 month minus 1 day
penicillin G potassium (aqueous)	250,000 units/mL	7 days minus 1 day
phenobarbital	65 mg/mL	1 month minus 1 day
phenobarbital dilution	10 mg/mL dilution	7 days
tobramycin	10 mg/mL (pediatric) 40 mg/mL (adult)	4 days minus 1 day
vancomycin	50 mg/mL	4 days minus 1 day
candida albicans antigen skin test	0.1 mL	1 month
mumps antigen skin test	0.1 mL	1 month
diptheria-tetanus-pertussis vaccine	0.5 mL	1 month
glycerin USP 99% (must be autoclaved)	2 mL	3 months

TABLE 9.5 Adult Pharmacy Nutrition Supply List

amino acids 8.5%	potassium phosphate 4.4 mEq/mL
dextrose 50%	potassium chloride 2 mEq/mL
dextrose 40%	potassium acetate 2 mEq/mL
dextrose 20%	magnesium sulfate 4.06 mEq/mL
lipids 20%	calcium gluconate 0.47 mEq/mL
lipids 10%	MVI (multivitamins)
sterile water	trace elements—4
sodium chloride 4 mEq/mL	heparin (beef) 1000 units/mL
sodium acetate 2 mEq/mL	sterile empty IV bags
sodium phosphate 4 mEq/mL	

TABLE 9.6 Neonatal Pharmacy Nutrition Supply List

TrophAmine 6%	potassium chloride 2 mEq/mL
dextrose 50%	potassium acetate 2 mEq/mL
lipids 20%	magnesium sulfate 4.06 mEq/mL
sterile water	calcium gluconate 0.47 mEq/mL
sodium chloride 4 mEq/mL	pediatric multivitamins
sodium acetate 2 mEq/mL	neonatal trace elements
sodium phosphate 4 mEq/mL	heparin (beef) 1000 units/mL
potassium phosphate 4.4 mEq/mL	sterile empty IV bags

PUZZLING TERMINOLOGY

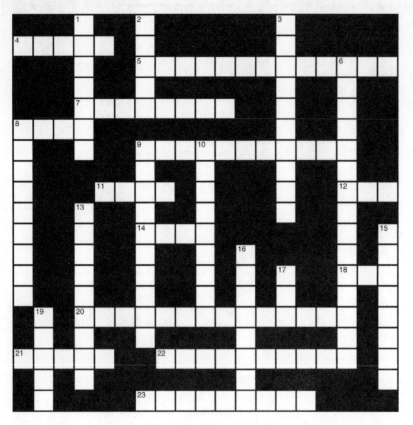

Down

1. documentation that provides the information necessary to prepare unit doses

2. independent, not-for-profit group that sets the standards by which quality of healthcare is measured and accredits hospitals according to those standards

3. one who comes to the hospital for treatment but then returns home

6. drugs being used in clinical trials that have not yet been approved for use in the general population, or drugs used for nonapproved indications

8. list of approved drugs available through a hospital pharmacy

9. ongoing study of drug usage patterns and costs within a hospital or other institution

10. one who stays in a hospital overnight for some time

13. precautions followed in healthcare settings to prevent infection as a result of exposure to blood or other bodily fluids

15. one aspect of prescription services that is reviewed during a quality assurance check

16. list of drugs and doses developed and approved by a physician for use by a nurse or pharmacist in the absence of the physician

17. hospital committee that reviews, approves, and revises the hospital's formulary

19. stock of medicatons kept on each nursing unit

Across

4. used needle; a source of infection

5. stamp of approval of the quality of services of a hospital by JCAHO

7. consent that is given after gaining a full understanding of the situation

8. complete list of all current medications for all hospital patients, used to create a unit dose profile

9. useful

11. medications that are to be administered immediately

12. hospital committee that ensures that patients using investigational drugs or procedures receive appropriate protection

14. dose of a drug prepackaged for a single administration to a particular patient at a particular time

18. hospital committee that provides leadership in relation to infection control techniques

20. restoration to a former condition

21. specially formulated parenteral solution that provides for nutritional needs intravenously

22. infection acquired by patients when they are in the hospital

23. minipharmacy located on a nursing unit of the hospital

Infection Control and Safe Handling of Hazardous Agents

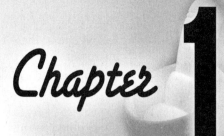

Chapter 10

IN THE LAB

The following lab activities should be carried out in the appropriate laboratory facility under supervision of your instructor.

Aseptic Technique

Hand Washing

Complete the following activity to learn about commonly accepted methods for disinfecting hands and to make yourself more conscious of the hands as a likely means for transfer of disease-causing microorganisms. This exercise also demonstrates the effectiveness of various materials and length of scrubbing for reducing skin surface bacterial numbers.

Supplies

- nutrient agar plates
- hand soap (Group 1)
- iodine-based disinfectant (Group 2) (Other scrub soaps may be substituted for students who are allergic to iodine.)
- alcohol wipes (Group 3)
- hand brushes
- sterile hand towels (optional)
- sterile cotton swabs
- sterile nutrient broth

Procedure

Students should work in groups of four. One student in each group acts as the control and should culture and swab an unwashed hand before streaking an agar plate. Each of the other three students should clean their hands using one of the techniques listed in Part 1 (page 130). Then complete the steps listed in Part 2.

Part 1

Follow *one* of these hand-washing procedures, as assigned to you by your instructor:

- Group 1: Wash your hands with soap and running water. Dry with a sterile towel.
- Group 2: Scrub your hands with a sterile hand brush and an iodine-based disinfectant for an assigned time. Dry your hands with a sterile towel.
- Group 3: Clean your hands with an alcohol wipe. Air-dry your hands.

Part 2

Inoculate the control plate. This plate will serve as one control in your experiment.

1. Wet the swab with sterile water or sterile nutrient broth.
2. Rub the swab over the hand.
3. Rub the swab lightly over the nutrient agar plate. Be careful not to tear the agar when inoculating it.
4. Label the plate with your group number, method, and time of washing; then inoculate a culture plate, following the steps outlined previously.

Part 3

Allow the culture plates to incubate at room temperature or in a slightly warm environment for at least 48 hours. Record the results of your test and those done by other students in your class.

Evaluation

Write a report summarizing your observations. Consider the following questions:

1. Which of the hand-washing techniques was most effective in decontaminating the hands? _____

    _____

    _____

    _____

2. What differences did you notice in the amount of culture produced using different lengths of time for scrubbing? _____

    _____

    _____

    _____

IV TPN Preparation

Your instructor will divide the class into groups. Using aseptic technique in a laminar airflow hood, add some vitamins and trace elements to a TPN solution provided. Let the instructor watch your technique.

Chemotherapy

Reconstitution and Sterile Preparation

Chemotherapy has its own special procedures and techniques. These exercises include chemo orders in which you will use Table 10.1, Chemotherapy Preparation and Dispensing Guidelines (pages 140–143), to answer questions concerning each order. A label is then to be written for each order. A drug not listed on the table will require a reference search.

1.

✓	START HERE →	DATE 2/25/XX	TIME 0800	PROFILED BY:	FILLED BY:	CHECKED BY:	PATIENT NAME AND I.D.

Please give thiotepa 15 mg at 1100 today

Dr. G. Jones

Knightley, Lisa 743125 Room 681

a. With what is this reconstituted? _____

_____

b. What is the vial concentration? _____

_____

c. What fluid is it diluted in for dispensing? _____

_____

d. How long is this to be infused? _____

_____

e. How long before this expires? _____

_____

f. Create a label and indicate special labeling requirements.

Mt. Hope Pharmacy Services

Patient: _____ ID. No._____ Rm. No. _____

Prepared: _____ Date:_____

Expiration: _____ By: _____

2.

(✓)	START HERE →	DATE 2/25/XX	TIME 1000		PROFILED BY:	FILLED BY:	CHECKED BY:	PATIENT NAME AND I.D.

cisplatin 45 mg dose to start today

Dr. Smith

Boyd, Franklin
387216
Room 672

a. With what is this reconstituted? _____

_____

b. What is the vial concentration? _____

_____

c. What fluid is it diluted in for dispensing? _____

_____

d. How long is this to be infused? _____

_____

e. How long before this expires? _____

_____

f. Create a label and indicate special labeling requirements.

Mt. Hope Pharmacy Services

Patient: _____ ID. No._____ Rm. No. _____

Prepared: _____ Date:_____

Expiration: _____ By: _____

3.

(✓)	START HERE ➡	DATE 2/10/XX	TIME 2040	PROFILED BY:	FILLED BY:	CHECKED BY:	PATIENT NAME AND I.D.

asparaginase 8000 units IV
1100

Dr. Holmes

Patient name column (vertical): Stevens, Robert 387317 Room 671

a. With what is this reconstituted? _____

_____

b. What is the vial concentration? _____

_____

c. What fluid is it diluted in for dispensing? _____

_____

d. How long is this to be infused? _____

_____

e. How long before this expires? _____

_____

f. Create a label and indicate special labeling requirements.

Mt. Hope Pharmacy Services

Patient: _____ ID. No._____ Rm. No. _____

Prepared: _____ Date:_____

Expiration: By:

4.

(✓)	START HERE	DATE 2/12/XX	TIME 0915	PROFILED BY:	FILLED BY:	CHECKED BY:	PATIENT NAME AND I.D.
							Hillary, Becky *3863* *Room 241*
		cyclophosphamide 1 g AM					
			Dr. Ledbetter				

a. With what is this reconstituted? _____

_____

b. What is the vial concentration? _____

_____

c. What fluid is it diluted in for dispensing? _____

_____

d. How long is this to be infused? _____

_____

e. How long before this expires? _____

_____

f. Create a label and indicate special labeling requirements.

Mt. Hope Pharmacy Services
Patient: _____ ID. No._____ Rm. No. _____
Prepared: _____ Date:_____
Expiration: By:

5.

✓	START HERE →	DATE 3/15/XX	TIME 1040	PROFILED BY:	FILLED BY:	CHECKED BY:	PATIENT NAME AND I.D.
							Singer, Gloria 38640 Room 221

Velban 15 mg PM

Dr. Haygood

a. With what is this reconstituted? _____

_____

b. What is the vial concentration? _____

_____

c. What fluid is it diluted in for dispensing? _____

_____

d. How long is this to be infused? _____

_____

e. How long before this expires? _____

_____

f. Create a label and indicate special labeling requirements.

Mt. Hope Pharmacy Services

Patient: _____   ID. No._____   Rm. No. _____

Prepared: _____   Date:_____

Expiration: _____   By: _____

6.

(✓)	START → HERE	DATE 4/20/XX	TIME 2350	PROFILED BY:	FILLED BY:	CHECKED BY:	PATIENT NAME AND I.D.
	bleomycin 15 units 1400						
	Dr. Fellows						

Patient name and I.D.: Mason, George 38641 Room 222

a. With what is this reconstituted? _____

_____

b. What is the vial concentration? _____

_____

c. What fluid is it diluted in for dispensing? _____

_____

d. How long is this to be infused? _____

_____

e. How long before this expires? _____

_____

f. Create a label and indicate special labeling requirements.

Mt. Hope Pharmacy Services

Patient: _____ ID. No._____ Rm. No. _____

Prepared: _____ Date:_____

Expiration: _____   By: _____

---

7. Use the following order for this practice on how to properly prepare a chemotherapy admixture:

(✓)	START → HERE	DATE 2/15/XX	TIME 1100	PROFILED BY:	FILLED BY:	CHECKED BY:	PATIENT NAME AND I.D.
							Lee, Wanda 36521 Room 1162
	Prepare Taxol 15 mg dose in D5W to make a final concentration of 0.3 mg/mL						
		Dr. Smith					

Use correct vertical airflow hood technique, and gather all materials needed to prepare before entering the hood. Your instructor will provide the Taxol drug.

a. Show calculations.

b. Prepare a label for this chemotherapy admixture.

> **Mt. Hope Pharmacy Services**
>
> Patient: _____   ID. No._____   Rm. No. _____
>
> Prepared: _____   Date:_____
>
>
>
>
>
>
> Expiration: _____   By:

Cytotoxic Materials Spill

This activity will simulate a hazardous materials spill (liquid, solid, or both). You will prepare for cleanup and handle the disposal in "appropriately labeled" containers. The full procedure for management of this type of incident will be covered.

1. Your instructor will simulate a spill that has occurred outside the biologic safety cabinet. Use the following chart to practice the procedural steps for cleaning up the spill:

	Activity	Check If Complete
1.	Place a warning sign and restrict access to the area.	
2.	Put on appropriate equipment (e.g., gown, gloves, respirator, and goggles).	
3.	Contain spill from the edges. Lay on spill pads. Check for splashes.	
4.	Scoop solids (e.g., glass).	
5.	Dispose of materials in appropriate containers. Confirm that containers are labeled.	
6.	Rinse the area with water.	
7.	Document the incident using the report form below.	

MT. HOPE HOSPITAL
CYTOTOXIC AND HAZARDOUS MATERIALS INCIDENT REPORT

Date: **Time**   **Dept.**

Person/persons Involved   **Sex**   **Date of birth**
Name:

Home Address   **Phone**

Sex   **Date of birth**
Name:

Home Address   **Phone**

Witness:

Description of Incident:

Agent and Amount of Spill:

Actions Taken:

Was Medical Treatment Necessary?
If Yes, Physician Name and Address:

Diagnosis:

Follow-up:

Suggestions for Prevention of Future Incidences:
Signature: _____
Title: **Date:**

2. Assume an accidental contact occurred to the back of your left hand while cleaning up the spill. Use the following chart to practice the procedural steps for attending to this incident:

	Activity	Check if Complete
1.	Remove gloves.	
2.	Wash with soap and water.	
3.	Request a physician examination.	
4.	Document the incident using the report form below.	

MT. HOPE HOSPITAL
CYTOTOXIC AND HAZARDOUS MATERIALS INCIDENT REPORT

Date: Time   Dept.

Person/persons Involved   Sex   Date of birth
Name:

Home Address   Phone

Sex   Date of birth
Name:

Home Address   Phone

Witness:

Description of Incident:

Agent and Amount of Spill:

Actions Taken:

Was Medical Treatment Necessary?
If Yes, Physician Name and Address:

Diagnosis:

Follow-up:

Suggestions for Prevention of Future Incidences:
Signature: _____
Title: Date:

TABLE 10.1 Chemotherapy Preparation and Dispensing Guidelines

Agent	Reconstitution	Dilution for Dispensing	Auxiliary Information
asparaginase (Elspar)	10,000 unit vial IM: add 1 mL NS (10,000 units/mL) IV: add 5 mL NS (2000 units/mL)	IM:* final concentration to be 10,000 units/mL in syringe IV push: final concentration to be 2000 units/mL in syringe IV infusion: place dose in 50 mL (NS only), infuse over 30 minutes or more	expiration: 8 hr at room temperature do not shake vial not stable in D_5W
bleomycin (Blenoxane)	15 unit vial add 1.5 mL SWFI (10/mL)	SC, IM: final concentration to be 100 mL in syringe IV push: final concentration to be 100 mL in syringe IV infusion:* place dose in 50 mL (D_5W, NS), infuse over 15 minutes or more	expiration: 24 hr at room temperature dispensed in glass; 1 hr dispensed in PVC container
carboplatin (Paraplatin)	50, 150, and 450 mg vials add 5, 15, 45 mL SWFI respectively (10 mg/mL)	IV infusion:* place dose in 100 mL (D_5W, NS), infuse over 30 minutes or more	expiration: 8 hr at room temperature
carmustine (BiCNU)	100 mg vial see vial for reconstitution*	IV infusion:* dose less than 20 mg, place dose in 100 mL (D_5W, NS); dose = 20–100 mg, place dose in 250 mL (D_5W, NS); dose greater than 100 mg, place dose in 500 mL (D_5W, NS)	expiration: 8 hr at room temperature dispense in glass protect from light must be diluted IV push not recommended
cisplatin (Platinol)	10 and 50 mg vials add 10 mL and 50 mL SWFI respectively (1 mg/mL) also forms an NS concentration because of NaCl present in vials	IV infusion:* dose less than 50 mg, place dose in 250 mL (NS, ½NS, ¼NS, D_5NS, D_5½NS, D_5¼NS); dose greater than 50 mg, place dose in 500 mL (NS, ½NS, ¼NS, D_5NS, D_5½NS, D_5¼NS); infuse over 2 hr or more	expiration: 24 hr at room temperature at least ¼NS must be present for stability do not refrigerate avoid aluminum needles
cyclophosphamide (Cytoxan)	100, 200, 500 mg vials add 5, 10, 25 mL SWFI respectively (20 mg/mL)	IV push: concentration to be 20 mg/mL in syringe IV infusion:* dose less than 500 mg, place dose in 50 mL (D_5W, NS); dose = 500 mg–1 g, place dose in 100 mL; dose greater than 1 g, place dose in 250 mL (D_5W, NS); infuse at 200 mg/hr or less	expiration: 24 hr at room temperature
cytarabine or ARA-C (Cytosar-U)	IV: 100 mg vial, add 5 mL SWFI (20 mg/mL); 500 mg vial, add 10 mL SWFI (50 mg/mL) SC, IM: 100 mg vial, add 1 mL SWFI (100 mg/mL)	SC, IM: concentration to be 100 mg/mL in syringe IM push: concentration to be 20 mg/mL in syringe or 50 mg/mL in syringe as per vial used	expiration: 24 hr at room temperature do not refrigerate call for specific dispensing guidelines for pediatric patient if not given
dacarbazine (DTIC-Dome)	200 mg vial see vial for reconstitution*	IV infusion:* dose less than 100 mg, place dose in 100 mL (D_5W, NS); dose 100–200 mg, place dose in 250 mL (D_5W, NS); dose greater than 200 mg, place dose in 500 mL; infuse over 30 minutes or more	expiration: 8 hr at room temperature protect from light avoid extravasation

(continues)

*Dispensing format unless otherwise stated per doctor's order or written request for nursing staff.

TABLE 10.1 (*CONTINUED*)

Agent	Reconstitution	Dilution for Dispensing	Auxiliary Information
dactinomycin or actinomycin-D (Cosmegen)	0.5 mg vial see vial for reconstitution*	IV push:* reconstitute to be 0.5 mg/mL in syringe IV infusion: place dose in 50 mL (D$_5$W, NS), infuse over 15 minutes or more	expiration: 24 hr at room temperature avoid extravasation
daunorubicin hydrochloride (Cerubidine)	see vial for reconstitution* add 4 mL SWFI (5 mg/mL)	IV push:* concentration to be 5 mg/mL in syringe IV infusion: place dose in 50 mL (D$_5$W, NS)	expiration: 24 hr at room temperature avoid extravasation
doxorubicin (Adriamycin)	see vial for reconstitution*	IV push:* concentration to be 2 mg/mL in syringe IV infusion: dose less than 50 mg, place dose in 50 mL (D$_5$W, NS); dose greater than 50 mg, place dose in 100 mL (D$_5$W, NS); infuse over 15 minutes or more	expiration: 24 hr at room temperature protect from light avoid extravasation call for specific dispensing guidelines for pediatric patient if not given
etoposide or VP-16 (Vepesid)	see vial for reconstitution*	IV infusion:* dose less than 100 mg, place dose in 250 mL (D$_5$W, NS); dose 100–200 mg, place dose in 500 mL (D$_5$W, NS); concentration less than 0.4 mg/mL; infuse over at least 60 minutes	expiration: for concentration less than 0.4 mg/mL, 48 hr at room temperature; for concentration = 0.4 mg/mL–0.6 mg/mL, 8 hr at room temperature; for concentration greater than 0.6 mg/mL, 2 hr at room temperature
floxuridine (FUDR)	500 mg vial add 5 mL SWFI (100 mg/mL)	IV infusion:* place dose in 250 mL (D$_5$W, NS), infuse over 60 minutes or more	expiration: 24 hr at room temperature do not refrigerate, but refrigerate reconstituted vials up to 2 hr
fluorouracil or 5-FU (Adrucil)	see vial for reconstitution*	IV push (not typical): concentration to be 50 mg/mL in syringe IV infusion: dose less than 1200 mg, place dose in 50 mL (D$_5$W, NS); dose = 1200–2500 mg, place dose in 100 mL (D$_5$W, NS); dose greater than 2500 mg, place dose in 250 mL (D$_5$W, NS); infuse 15 minutes or more	expiration: 24 hr at room temperature do not refrigerate if IV push ordered, ask for clarification because most 5-FU is given by continuous infusion in LVPs
ifosfamide (Ifex)	1 g vial add 20 mL SWFI (50 mg/mL)	IV push: concentration to be 50 mg/mL in syringe IV infusion:* dose less than 1 g, place dose in 100 mL (D$_5$W, NS); dose = 1–3 g, place dose in 250 mL (D$_5$W, NS); dose greater than 3 g, place dose in 500 mL (D$_5$W, NS); infuse over 30 minutes or more	expiration: 24 hr at room temperature
mechlorethamine or nitrogen mustard (Mustargen)	see vial for reconstitution*	dispense vial with nonbacteriostaic NS, and instruct nurse to mix only before administration	expiration: 30 minutes at room temperature avoid extravasation to be mixed on floor before use

(continues)

*Dispensing format unless otherwise stated per doctor's order or written request for nursing staff.

TABLE 10.1 *(CONTINUED)*

Agent	Reconstitution	Dilution for Dispensing	Auxiliary Information
methotrexate or MTX	see vial for reconstitution*	IV push: concentration to be 25 mg/mL in syringe IV infusion:* dose less than 500 mg, place dose 50 mL (D$_5$W, NS); dose = 500–1000 mg, place dose in 250 mL (D$_5$W, NS); dose greater than 1000 mg, place dose in 250 mL (D$_5$W, NS); infuse over 30 minutes or more	expiration: 24 hr at room temperature
mitomycin or mitomycin-C (Mutamycin)	see vial for reconstitution*	IV push:* concentration to be 0.5 mg/mL in syringe IV infusion: place dose in 50 mL (NS only), infuse over 15 minutes or more	expiration: 12 hr at room temperature avoid extravasation do not dilute in D$_5$W protect from light
mitoxantrone (Novantrone)	see vial for reconstitution*	IV infusion: place dose in 50 mL (D$_5$W, NS); infuse over 15 minutes or more; to be mixed on floor before use	expiration: 24 hr at room temperature IV push not recommended
plicamycin or mithramycin (Mithracin)	see vial for reconstitution*	IV infusion:* dose less than 2.5 mg, place dose in 500 mL (D$_5$W, NS); dose greater than 2.5 mg, place dose in 1000 mL (D$_5$W, NS); infuse over 4–6 hr	expiration: 24 hr at room temperature avoid extravasation
thiotepa	15 mg vial add 1.5 mL SWFI (10 mg/mL)	IV push:* concentration to be 10 mg/mL in syringe IV infusion: place dose in 50 mL (D$_5$W, NS), infuse over 15 minutes or more	expiration: 24 hr at room temperature
vinblastine (Velban)	10 mg vial add 10 mL NS (1 mg/mL)	IV push:* concentration to be 1 mg/mL in syringe IV infusion: place dose in 50 mL (D$_5$W, NS), infuse over 15 minutes or more	expiration: 24 hr at room temperature protect from light avoid extravasation
vincristine (Oncovin)	see vial for reconstitution*	IV push:* concentration to be 1 mg/mL in syringe IV infusion: place dose in 50 mL (D$_5$W, NS), infuse over 15 minutes or before	expiration: 24 hr at room temperature protect from light avoid extravasation

*Dispensing format unless otherwise stated per doctor's order or written request for nursing staff.

PUZZLING TERMINOLOGY

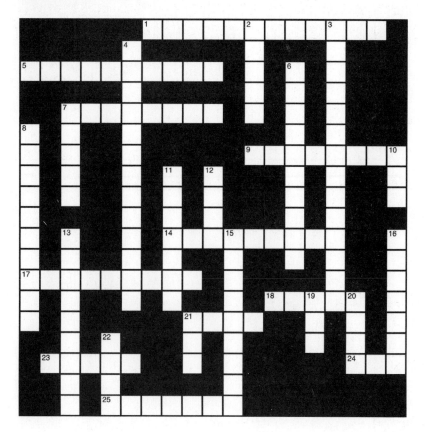

Across

1. chemical applied to an object or topically to the body for sterilization purposes

5. laminar airflow hood used to prepare IV drug admixtures, nutrition solutions, and other parenteral products aseptically

7. laminar airflow hood used to prepare hazardous drugs, especially cytotoxic drugs, aseptically

9. single-cell organisms that inhabit water and soil

14. microorganisms that cause infection

17. hazardous chemicals or drugs that must be handled and prepared with extra precautions

18. method of contamination that is the most common and the easiest to prevent

21. theory that microorganisms cause diseases

23. droplets that often contain harmful microorganisms

24. heat sterilization technique that is impractical for many substances but can be used to dispose of contaminated objects

25. absence of disease-causing microorganisms

Down

2. parasites on living organisms that feed on dead organic material and reproduce through spores

3. cancer-fighting drugs that are considered cytotoxic materials

4. introduction of harmful bacteria or other undesirable elements onto a sterile object or device or into a sterile solution

6. sterile products that are prepared outside the pharmaceutical manufacturer's facility

7. minute infectious agent that does not have all the components of a cell and thus can replicate only within a living host cell

8. sterilization that is accomplished by filtration

10. method of contamination that is controlled through the use of laminar airflow hoods

11. technique in which sterile products and devices are manipulated so as to avoid introducing pathogens or disease-causing organisms

12. sterilization technique that is readily available, effective, economical, and easily controlled

13. device that generates heat and pressure to sterilize

15. materials that require special handling and preparation

16. aspect of care that pharmacies must ensure through a formal feedback program

19. agency that has developed the guidelines used as accreditation standards for the preparation of parenteral products

20. special cabinet used to prepare parenteral drugs safely and aseptically

22. filter used with laminar airflow hoods to remove particulate matter larger than 0.3 micron

Preparing Sterile Intravenous Products

Chapter **11**

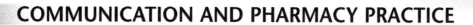

COMMUNICATION AND PHARMACY PRACTICE

1. A chemical sterilizer, an antiseptic, or a disinfectant can be used to kill germs. Where and in what manner is each used? _____

   _____

   _____

2. You have just been assigned to demonstrate cleaning the laminar airflow hood to a new employee. Describe the process and create a short list of "rules" that should be followed. _____

   _____

   _____

3. Describe what types of prescription products are prepared in a vertical laminar airflow hood and a horizontal airflow hood. _____

   _____

   _____

4. Label the parts of the syringe.

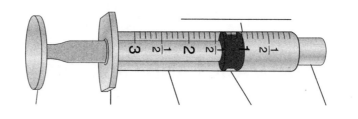

5. Label the parts of the needle.

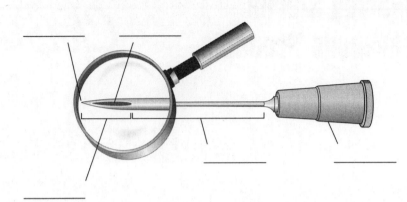

6. Label the parts of the IV administration set and IV bag.

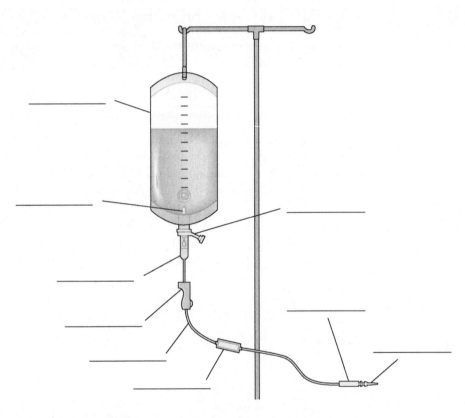

MATHEMATICS AND LAB REVIEW

For these exercises, use appropriate methods of measuring and calculating to arrive at correct answers. Refer to the reconstitutions chart (Table 9.3, pages 125–126) or consult the *Handbook on Injectable Drugs* to determine appropriate answers. Refer to Chapter 5 for basic math review if necessary.

1. Recall that a syringe is considered accurate to half the smallest measurement mark on its barrel. Read the volumes on the following syringes, and write the correct measurements on the lines provided.

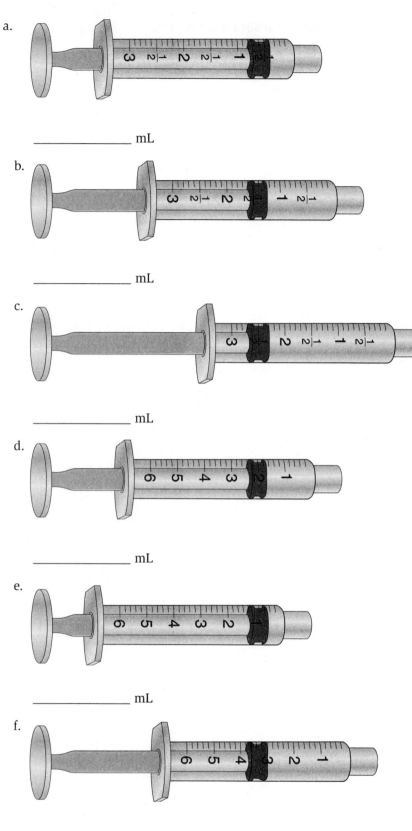

a. _____ mL

b. _____ mL

c. _____ mL

d. _____ mL

e. _____ mL

f. _____ mL

2. Convert the following times of day:

Clock Time	Military Time
9:05 AM	a. _____
b. _____	1653
c. _____	218
4:20 PM	d. _____
12:01 AM	e. _____
f. _____	0010

3. How many milligrams are in 100 mL of a 0.9% solution?

   _____

4. How many grams are in 2 L of a 5% solution of dextrose?

   _____

5. If a 1 L IV is running at a rate of 50 mL/hr, how many bags will be needed for a 24-hour period?

   _____

6. An IV is running at 125 mL/hr on a 10-drop set.

   a. What is the drip rate in gtt/min?

      _____

   b. How often will the bag need to be changed?

      _____

7. An order is written for 30 mEq KCl in 1 L $D_5\frac{1}{2}$ NS. The IV is run at 150 mL/hr.

   a. Is this a large volume?

      _____

   b. A stock bottle of KCl has 2 mEq/mL. How many milliliters of KCl will be needed for this order?

      _____

   c. How long will one bag last?

      _____

   d. How many bags will be needed?

      _____

8. An order reads: "Give Rocephin 0.5 g IV q24h."

a. Is this a large volume or minibag?

_____

b. What size bag will be needed?

_____

c. How many milliliters of Rocephin will be needed? Start with a 1 g vial that needs reconstitution.

_____

d. How many bags will be needed every 24 hours?

_____

9. Refer to this label to answer the following questions:

```
┌─────────────────────────────────────────────────┐
│            Mt. Hope Pharmacy Services             │
│                                                   │
│  Patient: COLMAN, SHERRY      ID. No. 024371     Rm. No. 541-1 │
│                                                   │
│  Prepared: 1050               Date: 10/15/XX     │
│                                                   │
│                 Rate: OVER 60 MIN                 │
│     SOD CHLORIDE 0.9%  100 ML                     │
│     AMPICILLIN/SULBACTUM                          │
│                                                   │
│          *REFRIGERATE*                            │
│                                                   │
│                                                   │
│     AS: UNASYN                                    │
│     FREQ: Q6H                                     │
│                                                   │
│  Expiration: 10/18/XX  1050           By:        │
└─────────────────────────────────────────────────┘
```

a. For what is the drug used?

_____

b. How many milliliters are used to reconstitute a 3 g vial of Unasyn?

_____

c. What is the resulting concentration?

_____

d. If kept refrigerated, how long until it expires?

_____

e. How many bags will be sent in a 24-hour period?

_____

10. Refer to this label to answer the following questions. *Note:* KCl has 2 mEq/mL and sodium bicarbonate has 1 mEq/mL.

Mt. Hope Pharmacy Services

Patient: BROWN, ROBERT   **ID. No.** 035481   **Rm. No.** 649-1

Prepared: 1330   **Date:** 03/25/XX

Rate: 85 ML/HR
DEXTROSE 5% W1/2NS 1000 ML
POTASSIUM CHLORIDE 30 mEq
SODIUM BICARBONATE 20 mEq

AS: IV FLUSH

FREQ: Q12H

Expiration: 03/26/XX   1330   **By:**

---

a. How many milliliters of KCl and sodium bicarbonate will be needed?

_____

b. How long will one bag last?

_____

c. How many bags will be needed every 24 hours?

_____

11. Refer to this label to answer the following questions. Note that heparin has 10,000 units/mL and aminophylline has 500 mg/20 mL.

Mt. Hope Pharmacy Services

Patient: HARE, ROGER   **ID. No.** 035481   **Rm. No.** 420

Prepared: 1440   **Date:** 06/21/XX

Rate: 125 ML/HR
1000 ML DEXTROSE 5% LACTATED RINGER'S
HEPARIN 7500 UNITS
AMINOPHYLLINE 400 MG

FREQ: Q8H

Expiration: 06/22/XX   1440   **By:**

---

a. How many milliliters of heparin and aminophylline will be needed?

_____

b. How long will a bag last?

_____

c. How many units/mL of heparin are in the bag?

_____

d. What is the mg/mL of aminophylline in the bag?

_____

12. Prepare a label for an order that reads:

(✓)	START HERE →	DATE 1/28/XX	TIME 1000	PROFILED BY:	FILLED BY:	CHECKED BY:	PATIENT NAME AND I.D.
							Thomas, D. E. 145678 Room 432
	give Cefobid 1 g q12h x 3 days						

Mt. Hope Pharmacy Services

Patient: _____ ID. No. _____ Rm. No. _____

Prepared: _____ Date: _____

Expiration: _____   By: _____

Following aseptic technique, prepare the previous order. When you have completed the order, ask your instructor to check your work.

13. Prepare a label for an order that reads:

(✓)	START → HERE	DATE 2/25/XX	TIME 2240	PROFILED BY:	FILLED BY:	CHECKED BY:	PATIENT NAME AND I.D.
							Tompkins, John 1567842 Room 306
		give Primaxin 500 mg q12h					

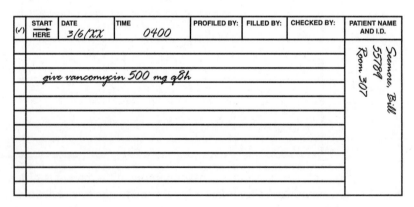

Mt. Hope Pharmacy Services

Patient: _____ ID. No._____ Rm. No. _____

Prepared: _____ Date:_____

Expiration: By:

14. Prepare a label for an order that reads:

(✓)	START → HERE	DATE 3/6/XX	TIME 0400	PROFILED BY:	FILLED BY:	CHECKED BY:	PATIENT NAME AND I.D.
							Seemore, Bill 55789 Room 307
		give vancomycin 500 mg q8h					

```
                    Mt. Hope Pharmacy Services
   Patient: _____   ID. No._____   Rm. No. _____

   Prepared: _____   Date:_____










   Expiration: _____                    By:
```

IN THE LAB

The following lab activities should be carried out in the appropriate laboratory facility under supervision of your instructor.

Small-Volume Parenterals (SVPs) (Minibags)

Read each medication order carefully and answer the questions related to that order. Consult the appropriate drug references, Table 9.1, Minibag Administration Protocol (pages 123–124), and Table 9.3, Reconstitutions (pages 125–126). (These tables will also be needed in other workbook exercises related to Chapter 11.)

1.

(✓)	START HERE	DATE	TIME	PROFILED BY:	FILLED BY:	CHECKED BY:	PATIENT NAME AND I.D.
	→	1/28/XX	1000				Robinson, Mary 1234567 Room 159
	Azactam 2 g q8h						
			Dr. Smith				

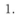

a. What is the use of the ordered medication?

_____

b. Is this an oral dose form?

_____

c. Over how long should this be infused?

_____

d. What size minibag should be used?

_____

e. How much diluent is needed?

_____

f. Prepare a label for this order.

```
┌─────────────────────────────────────────────────────────┐
│              Mt. Hope Pharmacy Services                  │
│                                                          │
│   Patient: _____  ID. No._____  Rm. No. ____ │
│                                                          │
│   Prepared: _____  Date:_____          │
│                                                          │
│                                                          │
│                                                          │
│                                                          │
│                                                          │
│                                                          │
│                                                          │
│                                                          │
│   Expiration:                              By:           │
│                                                          │
└─────────────────────────────────────────────────────────┘
```

2.

START HERE →	DATE 1/29/XX	TIME 2300	PROFILED BY:	FILLED BY:	CHECKED BY:	PATIENT NAME AND I.D.
						Robinson, Mary 1234567 Room 159
D/C Azactam start ampicillin 1 g q6h						
Smith, MD						

a. What is the use of the ordered medication?

_____

b. Is there an oral dose form for this medication?

_____

c. Over how long should this be infused?

_____

d. What size minibag should be used?

_____

e. How much diluent is needed?

_____

f. Prepare a label for this order.

```
┌──────────────────────────────────────────────────────────────┐
│                  Mt. Hope Pharmacy Services                  │
│                                                              │
│   Patient: _____  ID. No._____  Rm. No. _____  │
│                                                              │
│   Prepared: _____  Date:_____                  │
│                                                              │
│                                                              │
│                                                              │
│                                                              │
│                                                              │
│                                                              │
│                                                              │
│                                                              │
│   Expiration:                              By:               │
│                                                              │
└──────────────────────────────────────────────────────────────┘
```

3.

✓	START → HERE	DATE 2/15/XX	TIME 0400	PROFILED BY:	FILLED BY:	CHECKED BY:	PATIENT NAME AND I.D.
							Cacher, William 1234578 Room 204
		Amicar 3 g q12h					
			Dr. Cure				

a. What is the use of the ordered medication?

_____

b. Over how long should this be infused?

_____

c. What size minibag should be used?

_____

d. What fluid should be added?

_____

e. Should this be stored under refrigeration? If so, how long?

_____

f. Prepare a label for this order.

```
┌─────────────────────────────────────────────────────────────────┐
│                   Mt. Hope Pharmacy Services                      │
│                                                                   │
│   Patient: _____  ID. No._____  Rm. No. _____│
│                                                                   │
│   Prepared: _____  Date:_____         │
│                                                                   │
│                                                                   │
│                                                                   │
│                                                                   │
│                                                                   │
│                                                                   │
│                                                                   │
│                                                                   │
│                                                                   │
│                                                                   │
│   Expiration:                                    By:              │
└─────────────────────────────────────────────────────────────────┘
```

4.

(✓)	START ⟶ HERE	DATE 2/15/XX	TIME 1500	PROFILED BY:	FILLED BY:	CHECKED BY:	PATIENT NAME AND I.D.
							Crunch, Carolyn 1234572 Room 205
		ranitidine 25 mg q8h					
		Dr. Cure					

a. What is the use of the ordered medication?

_____

b. Is there an oral dose form of this medication?

_____

c. Over how long should this be infused?

_____

d. What size minibag should be used?

_____

e. Should this be stored under refrigeration? If so, how long?

_____

f. Prepare a label for this order.

```
┌──────────────────────────────────────────────────────────────┐
│                  Mt. Hope Pharmacy Services                    │
│                                                                │
│  Patient: _____      ID. No._____  Rm. No. ____ │
│                                                                │
│  Prepared: _____     Date:_____                │
│                                                                │
│                                                                │
│                                                                │
│                                                                │
│                                                                │
│                                                                │
│                                                                │
│                                                                │
│  Expiration:                                By:                │
└──────────────────────────────────────────────────────────────┘
```

Large-Volume Parenterals (LVPs)

Carefully read each medication order, and answer the questions related to that order.

1.

(✓)	START HERE	DATE 1/28/XX	TIME 2000	PROFILED BY:	FILLED BY:	CHECKED BY:	PATIENT NAME AND I.D.
							Robinson, Mary 1234567 Room 159

Put 20 mEq KCl in 1 L D5W at 100 mL/hr

Smith, MD

a. What size bag will be needed?

_____

b. What is the infusion rate?

_____

c. How many hours will one bag last?

_____

d. Prepare a label for the order.

```
┌─────────────────────────────────────────────────────────────┐
│                 Mt. Hope Pharmacy Services                  │
│                                                             │
│  Patient: _____    ID. No._____  Rm. No. ____ │
│                                                             │
│  Prepared: _____    Date:_____              │
│                                                             │
│                                                             │
│                                                             │
│                                                             │
│                                                             │
│                                                             │
│                                                             │
│                                                             │
│                                                             │
│                                                             │
│                                                             │
│  Expiration:                              By:               │
│                                                             │
└─────────────────────────────────────────────────────────────┘
```

2.

(✓)	START →HERE	DATE 1/29/XX	TIME 0900	PROFILED BY:	FILLED BY:	CHECKED BY:	PATIENT NAME AND I.D.
							Robinson, Mary 1234567 Room 159
	Change IVF to						
	20 mEq potassium chloride						
	2 g mag sulfate						
	in 1 L NS @ 100 mL/hr						
		Smith, MD					

a. What size bag will be needed?

_____

b. What is the infusion rate?

_____

c. How many hours will one bag last?

_____

d. Prepare a label for the order.

Mt. Hope Pharmacy Services

Patient: _____   ID. No._____   Rm. No. _____

Prepared: _____   Date:_____

Expiration: By:

3.

(✓)	START HERE ➡	DATE 2/15/XX	TIME 0945		PROFILED BY:	FILLED BY:	CHECKED BY:	PATIENT NAME AND I.D.
								Williams, Charlie
	L D₅W at 125 mL/hr							*1234528*
	NaCl at 5 mEq							*Room 411*
	mag sulfate 4 mEq							
	KCl 10 mEq							
	Dr. Lee Won							

a. What size of bag will be needed?

_____

b. What is the infusion rate?

_____

c. How many hours will one bag last?

_____

d. How many milliequivalents of electrolytes per milliliter are needed?

_____

e. Prepare a label for the order.

Mt. Hope Pharmacy Services

Patient: _____   ID. No._____   Rm. No. _____

Prepared: _____   Date:_____

Expiration: _____   By:

4.

✓	START HERE →	DATE 3/5/XX	TIME 1100	PROFILED BY:	FILLED BY:	CHECKED BY:	PATIENT NAME AND I.D.
							Neon. Agustina 1234857 Room 315
	D₅W 500 mL at 50 mL/hr						
	insulin 100 units						
		Dr. Liggett					

a. What size bag will be needed?

_____

b. What is the infusion rate?

_____

c. How many hours will one bag last?

_____

d. How many units of insulin are needed per milliliter?

_____

e. What special precautions should be taken when mixing and administering this medication?

_____

_____

f. Prepare a label for the order.

```
┌──────────────────────────────────────────────────┐
│            Mt. Hope Pharmacy Services             │
│                                                    │
│   Patient: _____  ID. No._____   Rm. No. _____  │
│                                                    │
│   Prepared: _____  Date:_____   │
│                                                    │
│                                                    │
│                                                    │
│                                                    │
│                                                    │
│                                                    │
│                                                    │
│   Expiration:                        By:           │
│                                                    │
└──────────────────────────────────────────────────┘
```

IV Labels

Carefully read these labels and answer the questions. For additional aseptic compounding experience, follow the instructions in exercise 5 on page 163. Prepare a label (page 164) and the admixture. Demonstrate all procedures and techniques for the instructor.

1.

```
┌──────────────────────────────────────────────────┐
│            Mt. Hope Pharmacy Services             │
│                                                    │
│   Patient:  MEEKS, AGNES      ID. No. 042311    Rm. No. 589-1  │
│                                                    │
│   Prepared:  0800             Date:  12/02/XX      │
│                                                    │
│              Rate: OVER 60 MIN                     │
│        SOD CHLORIDE 0.9%  100  ML                  │
│        IMIPENEM/CILASTATIN                         │
│                                                    │
│            *REFRIGERATE*                           │
│                                                    │
│                                                    │
│   AS:  PRIMAXIN                                     │
│   FREQ:  Q12H                                       │
│                                                    │
│   Expiration:  12/04/XX  0800            By:       │
│                                                    │
└──────────────────────────────────────────────────┘
```

a. Is this a minibag or large-volume preparation?

_____

b. Over how long will this drug be infused?

_____

c. How many times a day will the patient get this drug?

_____

2.

Mt. Hope Pharmacy Services

Patient: NEWTON, NANCY   **ID. No.** 033371   **Rm. No.** 510-2

Prepared: 1445   **Date:** 12/02/XX

Rate: 50 ML/HR
DEXTROSE 5% 1/2NS 1000 ML
POTASSIUM CHLORIDE 60 mEq

AS: PRIMAXIN

FREQ:

Expiration: 12/03/XX 1445   **By:**

a. Is this a minibag or large-volume preparation?

_____

b. What is the rate of infusion?

_____

c. How long will one bag last?

_____

3.

Mt. Hope Pharmacy Services

Patient: SPALDING, MICHELE   **ID. No.** 053481   **Rm. No.** 515-2

Prepared: 0600   **Date:** 12/02/XX

Rate: OVER 60 MIN
DEXTROSE 5% 250 ML
VANCOMYCIN HCL 1000 MG

AS: VANCOMYCIN

FREQ: Q12H

Expiration: 12/06/XX 0600   **By:**

a. Is this a minibag or large-volume preparation?

_____

b. Over how long will this drug be infused?

_____

c. How many times a day will the patient receive the medication?

_____

4.

```
┌─────────────────────────────────────────────────────────┐
│              Mt. Hope Pharmacy Services                  │
│                                                          │
│   Patient: TAYLOR, JAMES      ID. No. 066281   Rm. No. 327│
│                                                          │
│   Prepared:  1520             Date: 11/02/XX             │
│                                                          │
│                                                          │
│             Rate: 25  ML/HR                              │
│   DEXTROSE 5%  500  ML                                   │
│   HEPARIN SODIUM  1000  UNITS                            │
│                                                          │
│                                                          │
│                                                          │
│   AS:                                                    │
│   FREQ:                                                  │
│                                                          │
│   Expiration: 11/03/XX   1520             By:            │
└─────────────────────────────────────────────────────────┘
```

a. Is this a minibag or large-volume preparation?

_____

b. What is the rate of infusion?

_____

c. How long will one bag last?

_____

5. Read the following order:

(✓)	START HERE →	DATE 1/29/XX	TIME 0300	PROFILED BY:	FILLED BY:	CHECKED BY:	PATIENT NAME AND I.D.
							Jones, C. *782736* *Room 371*
		start Cefolid 1 g q12h					
			Smith, MD				

a. Prepare the medication. Make sure that as part of the preparation process, you wash your hands and clean the hood properly.

b. Prepare a label for the order.

```
┌─────────────────────────────────────────────────────┐
│              Mt. Hope Pharmacy Services               │
│  Patient: _____  ID. No._____  Rm. No. _____  │
│                                                       │
│  Prepared: _____   Date:_____     │
│                                                       │
│                                                       │
│                                                       │
│                                                       │
│                                                       │
│                                                       │
│                                                       │
│                                                       │
│                                                       │
│                                                       │
│                                                       │
│  Expiration: _____          By: _____   │
│                                                       │
└─────────────────────────────────────────────────────┘
```

Reconstitution and Protocol Charts

Use the information found in Table 9.1, Minibag Administration Protocol (pages 123–124), and Table 9.3, Reconstitutions (pages 125–126), to answer the following questions:

1. How many milliliters are used to reconstitute the following pharmaceuticals?

   a. Mandol 1 g _____

   b. Ticar 3 g _____

   c. Zinacef 1.5 g _____

2. What are the resulting concentrations?

   a. Mandol 1 g _____

   b. Ticar 3 g _____

   c. Zinacef 1.5 g _____

3. What type of fluid would be used to administer the medication, and how many milliliters would be needed?

   a. Mandol 1 g _____

   b. Ticar 3 g _____

   c. Zinacef 1.5 g _____

4. What length of infusion time would be printed on the label?

   a. Mandol 1 g _____

   b. Ticar 3 g _____

   c. Zinacef 1.5 g _____

5. What special information should be included on these medication labels?

   a. Septra_____

   b. furosemide _____

   c. Flagyl_____

Exercise 6 provides an opportunity to use medication charts, do appropriate calculations if necessary, gather materials, and prepare the admixture. (Preparing a label will be at the instructor's discretion.) Your instructor may wish to vary the drug strength, thus requiring a calculation and a variance in dose.

6. Gather the materials to make the following:

> R_x Unasyn 3 g q6h to start at 1200 today

    a. Reconstitute the vial and give the resulting concentration.

       _____

    b. What fluid volume will be used to reconstitute?

       _____

    c. In what fluid will the drug be placed and in what volume?

       _____

Exercises 7 and 8 offer additional opportunities to acquire information from orders, prepare labels, and compound the admixture.

7.

(✓)	START → HERE	DATE 2/4/XX	TIME 1100	PROFILED BY:	FILLED BY:	CHECKED BY:	PATIENT NAME AND I.D.
							Adams, Luke 38920 Room 411

hang aminophylline 250 mg in D₅W
500 mL to start now
infuse at 35 mL/hr

Dr. Grad

    a. Is this a large-volume parenteral or a minibag?

       _____

    b. What size bag is needed?

       _____

    c. How long will one bag last?

       _____

    d. How many bags (approximately) will be needed every 24 hours?

       _____

    e. Prepare this order.

f. Prepare a label.

```
┌─────────────────────────────────────────────────────┐
│              Mt. Hope Pharmacy Services             │
│                                                     │
│  Patient: _____  ID. No._____  Rm. No. _____  │
│                                                     │
│  Prepared: _____  Date:_____    │
│                                                     │
│                                                     │
│                                                     │
│                                                     │
│                                                     │
│                                                     │
│                                                     │
│                                                     │
│                                                     │
│                                                     │
│  Expiration:                          By:          │
└─────────────────────────────────────────────────────┘
```

8.

(✓)	START HERE ➡	DATE 2/4/XX	TIME 0900	PROFILED BY:	FILLED BY:	CHECKED BY:	PATIENT NAME AND I.D.
							Jones, Mary, 369752 Room 110-1
		start 1 L LR with 20 mEq KCl at 125 mL/hr					
		Dr. Grad					

a. Is this a large-volume parenteral or a minibag?

_____

b. What size bag is needed?

_____

c. How long will one bag last?

_____

d. How many bags (approximately) will be needed every 24 hours?

_____

e. Prepare this order.

f. Prepare a label.

```
┌─────────────────────────────────────────────────────────────────┐
│                   Mt. Hope Pharmacy Services                      │
│                                                                   │
│   Patient: _____  ID. No._____  Rm. No. _____ │
│                                                                   │
│   Prepared: _____  Date:_____          │
│                                                                   │
│                                                                   │
│                                                                   │
│                                                                   │
│                                                                   │
│                                                                   │
│                                                                   │
│                                                                   │
│                                                                   │
│                                                                   │
│   Expiration:                              By:                    │
│                                                                   │
└─────────────────────────────────────────────────────────────────┘
```

9.

(✓)	START HERE	DATE 6/20/XX	TIME 1100	PROFILED BY:	FILLED BY:	CHECKED BY:	PATIENT NAME AND I.D.
							Wisker, Tom 3275621 Room 722
		ampicillin 1.5 g q8h					
			Dr. Jitters				

a. What fluid will you use to reconstitute this order?

_____

b. How much fluid will you need to reconstitute this order?

_____

c. The pharmacy has 2 g and 10 g vials available. Which size vial will you use, and how much is drawn from that vial?

_____

d. What fluid is the drug mixed in for administration?

_____

e. What size bag should be used?

_____

f. How long should this be infused?

_____

g. What is the expiration time if stored under refrigeration?

_____

h. How many admixture solutions are to be prepared for 24 hours?

_____

i. Prepare a label.

```
┌─────────────────────────────────────────────────────────────┐
│                  Mt. Hope Pharmacy Services                  │
│                                                              │
│   Patient: _____   ID. No. _____  Rm. No. _____ │
│                                                              │
│   Prepared: _____   Date: _____         │
│                                                              │
│                                                              │
│                                                              │
│                                                              │
│                                                              │
│                                                              │
│                                                              │
│                                                              │
│                                                              │
│   Expiration:                              By:               │
│                                                              │
└─────────────────────────────────────────────────────────────┘
```

10.

(✓)	START HERE →	DATE	TIME		PROFILED BY:	FILLED BY:	CHECKED BY:	PATIENT NAME AND I.D.
		3/30/XX	0000					*Archie, Jennifer* *3274722* *Room 622*
		vancomycin 2 g q12h						
			Dr. Hess					

a. What fluid will you use to reconstitute this order?

_____

b. How much fluid will you need to reconstitute this order?

_____

c. The pharmacy has 5 g vials available. How much is drawn from the vial?

_____

d. What fluid is the drug mixed in for administration?

_____

e. What size bag should be used?

_____

f. How long should this be infused?

_____

g. What is the expiration time if stored under refrigeration?

_____

h. How many admixture solutions are to be prepared for 24 hours?

_____

i. Prepare a label.

```
┌─────────────────────────────────────────────────────────┐
│              Mt. Hope Pharmacy Services                  │
│                                                          │
│   Patient: _____  ID. No._____  Rm. No. _____ │
│                                                          │
│   Prepared: _____  Date:_____          │
│                                                          │
│                                                          │
│                                                          │
│                                                          │
│                                                          │
│                                                          │
│                                                          │
│   Expiration:                          By:               │
│                                                          │
└─────────────────────────────────────────────────────────┘
```

11.

(✓)	START HERE →	DATE 8/15/XX	TIME 1500	PROFILED BY:	FILLED BY:	CHECKED BY:	PATIENT NAME AND I.D.
							Markowicz, Margie 3365321 Room 481
	give Mefoxin 1.75 g q6h						
		Dr. Smith					

a. What fluid will you use to reconstitute this order?

_____

b. How much fluid will you need to reconstitute this order?

_____

c. The pharmacy has 1 g, 2 g, and 10 g vials available. Which size vial will you use and how much is drawn from that vial?

_____

d. What fluid is the drug mixed in for administration?

_____

e. What size bag should be used?

_____

f. How long should this be infused?

_____

g. What is the expiration time if stored under refrigeration?

_____

h. How many admixture solutions are to be prepared for 24 hours?

_____

i. Prepare a label.

```
┌─────────────────────────────────────────────────────────┐
│                Mt. Hope Pharmacy Services                 │
│                                                           │
│   Patient: _____  ID. No._____  Rm. No. _____ │
│                                                           │
│   Prepared: _____  Date:_____       │
│                                                           │
│                                                           │
│                                                           │
│                                                           │
│                                                           │
│                                                           │
│                                                           │
│                                                           │
│   Expiration:                              By:            │
└─────────────────────────────────────────────────────────┘
```

12.

(✓)	START HERE →	DATE	TIME	PROFILED BY:	FILLED BY:	CHECKED BY:	PATIENT NAME AND I.D.
		11/16/XX	1600				
							Bunker, Amy
	give nafcillin 1.5 g q8h						3333621
							Room 222
	Dr. W. Mark						

a. What fluid will you use to reconstitute this order?

_____

b. How much fluid will you need to reconstitute this order?

_____

c. The pharmacy has 500 mg and 1, 2, and 10 g vials available. Which size vial will you use, and how much is drawn from the vial?

_____

d. What fluid is the drug mixed in for administration?

_____

e. What size bag should be used?

_____

f. How long should this be infused?

_____

g. What is the expiration time if stored under refrigeration?

_____

h. How many admixture solutions are to be prepared for 24 hours?

_____

i. Prepare a label.

Mt. Hope Pharmacy Services		
Patient: _____	ID. No. _____	Rm. No. _____
Prepared: _____	Date: _____	
Expiration:	By:	

13.

(✓)	START HERE	DATE 2/2/XX	TIME 1000	PROFILED BY:	FILLED BY:	CHECKED BY:	PATIENT NAME AND I.D.
							Thomas, D. C. *368241* *Room 481*
	ranitidine 50 mg q12h						
		Will Romez, MD					

a. What fluid will you use to reconstitute this order?

_____

b. How much fluid will you need to reconstitute this order?

_____

c. The pharmacy has 50 mg vials available. How much is drawn from that vial?

_____

d. What fluid is the drug mixed in for administration?

_____

e. What size bag should be used?

_____

f. How long should this be infused?

_____

g. What is the expiration time if stored under refrigeration?

_____

h. How many admixture solutions are to be prepared for 24 hours?

_____

i. Prepare a label.

Mt. Hope Pharmacy Services

Patient: _____ ID. No._____ Rm. No. _____

Prepared: _____ Date:_____

Expiration: By:

14.

(✓)	START HERE	DATE 2/7/XX	TIME 0400	PROFILED BY:	FILLED BY:	CHECKED BY:	PATIENT NAME AND I.D.
							Peabody, Lester 4554322 Room 206
		1 L D5W infuse at 125 mL/hr					
		KCl 6 mEq					
		calcium gluconate 3 mEq					
		sodium acetate 4 mEq					
		heparin 1500 units					
		multivitamins 2 mL					
		Dr. Goodroot					

You have the following vials available:

KCl	2 mEq/mL
calcium gluconate	4.87 mEq/10 mL
sodium acetate	2 mEq/mL
heparin	10,000 units/mL
multivitamins	3 mL

a. What fluid will you use to reconstitute this order?

_____

b. What size bag should be used?

_____

c. Is this a large or small volume?

_____

d. How much of each drug will be drawn up?

    1) KCl_____

    2) calcium gluconate_____

    3) sodium acetate_____

    4) heparin _____

    5) multivitamins _____

e. How long will a bag run?

_____

f. If the first bag is hung at 0600, when is the next one due?

_____

g. How many bags are needed for 24 hours?

_____

h. What is the expiration in number of hours?

_____

i. Prepare a label.

Mt. Hope Pharmacy Services

Patient: _____   ID. No._____   Rm. No. _____

Prepared: _____   Date:_____

Expiration: By:

PUZZLING TERMINOLOGY

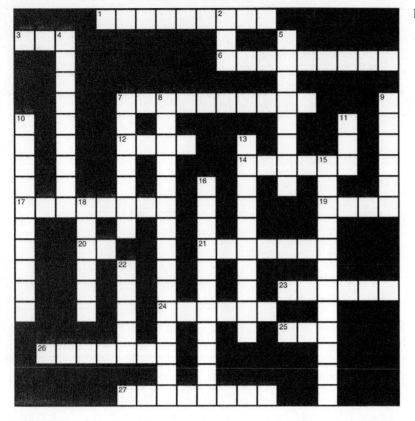

Down

2. IV infusion of more than 100 mL

4. small-volume parenteral admixture, often containing a medication, that is attached to an existing IV line

5. parenteral solution with the same number of particles as blood cells

7. the pressure produced by or associated with osmosis

8. millimole divided by its valence

9. device used to remove contaminants such as glass, paint, fibers, and rubber cores from IV fluids

10. type of injection port found on most IV administration sets

11. very fine catheter that is threaded through the peripheral vein into the subclavian vein

13. temperature scale that uses 32 degrees as the temperature at which water freezes and 212 degrees as the temperature at which water boils

15. breakdown or collapse of a vein that allows the drug to leak into tissues surrounding the catheter site, causing edema or tissue damage or both

16. dissolved mineral salt, found in IV fluids

18. single-dose drug container

22. another word for the bore of a catheter

Across

1. weight that is the sum of the atomic weights of all the atoms in one molecule of a compound

3. IV infusion of 100 mL or less

6. phosphorus-oxygen combination found in solution

7. amount of particulate per unit volume of a liquid preparation, measured in milliosmoles

12. measurement of an element equal to its atomic weight in grams

14. pH of less than 7

17. pH of more than 7

19. number of lumens in a catheter used to administer potentially incompatible drugs to the most ill patients

20. degree of acidity or alkalinity of a solution

21. catheter placed deep into a vein in the body

23. introducing a small chunk of the rubber closure into the solution while removing medication from a vial

24. weight of a single atom of an element compared with the weight of one atom of hydrogen

25. sterile, pyrogen-free, disposable equipment used to administer IV fluids

26. number that represents an element's capacity to combine to form a molecule of a stable compound

27. device inserted into veins for direct access to the blood vascular system

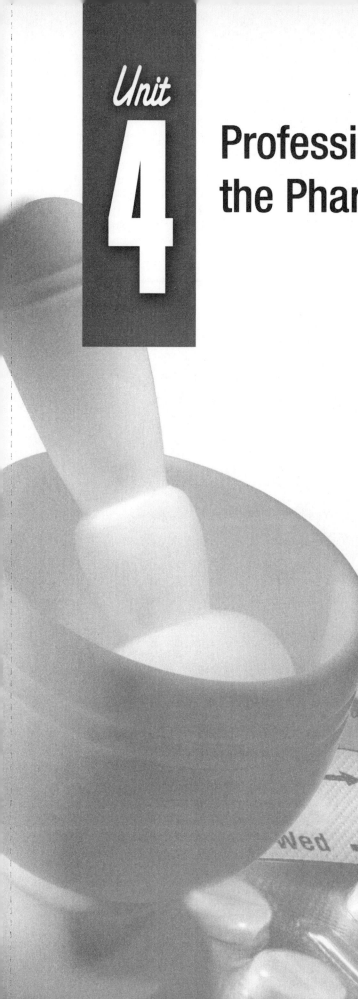

Unit 4

Professionalism in the Pharmacy

Medication Safety
by Jennifer Danielson

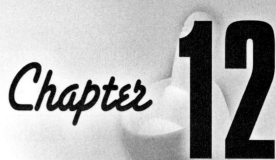

Chapter **12**

COMMUNICATION AND PHARMACY PRACTICE

1. Review Chapter 12 and Appendix E in the textbook, and answer the following questions about methods used to prevent medication errors:

    a. What are some of the most common errors that are made on prescriptions?

    _____

    b. When should the technician check to see if the correct drug is being used to fill a prescription?

    _____

    c. When should the pharmacist check to see if the correct drug is being used to fill a prescription?

    _____

    d. What math rules should be followed?

    _____

    e. What should be done if a prescriber error is found?

    _____

    f. Why is storage of medication an important issue to consider?

    _____

    g. What happens to the hard-copy prescription after the original fill date?

    _____

    h. What should be the final checkpoint?

    _____

2. Think about when a prescription is interpreted and entered into the computer. List three mistakes that can happen at this point and lead to a medication error, and describe the procedures that should be followed to prevent them.

    _____

    _____

    _____

---

3. Think about retrieving medication to fill a prescription. Name two mistakes that can happen at this point and lead to an incorrect selection error, and describe the procedures that should be followed to prevent them.

_____

_____

4. A patient comes to the counter with her prescription that was refilled yesterday. She states that the pills she was given do not look like the ones she normally gets and says she is worried that she has taken the wrong drug.

   a. What should you tell her, and what should you do in this situation? What questions will you have for her to begin with, and what will be your first course of action?

   _____

   _____

   b. Sometimes a medication error is suspected when the pharmacy has simply changed generic drug suppliers. The new generic product can look different from the previous product used to fill the prescription (i.e., it might be a different color, shape, or size); however, it may still be an appropriate generic substitution. How would your actions and words differ if the suspected error turned out to be an appropriate substitution versus an actual medication error?

   _____

   _____

WEB ACTIVITIES

Visit the Institute for Safe Medication Practices (ISMP) Web site, at www.ismp.org, and answer the following questions:

1. Locate two reports of an error made in the inpatient setting and two reports of an error made in the outpatient setting. Read about what happened and answer these questions: How did a technician contribute to each mistake made? How could a technician have helped the pharmacist (and other health-care professionals) avoid these errors?

2. Locate information on abbreviations that *should not* be used. Find three abbreviations that could easily be misread or misinterpreted on a physician's order, especially if faxed to the pharmacy; then find three more abbreviations that could easily be misinterpreted by a nurse administering medications.

3. Locate information on sound-alike, look-alike drug names. Find two examples in which confusing like drugs would cause potentially life-threatening consequences; then find two examples in which the consequences of switching like drugs would not be life-threatening and could be handled through referral to the pharmacist for counseling and education.

4. Locate the Medication Error Reporting Program (MERP). How is a report made? What information is contained in a MERP report?

PUZZLING TERMINOLOGY

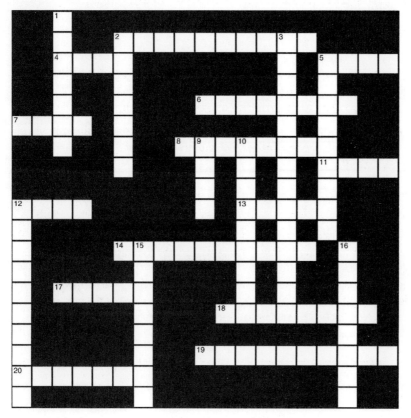

18. logical and systematic process used to help identify what, how, and why something happened

19. capacity for being read clearly

20. error that occurs when focus on a task is diverted elsewhere, allowing a mistake to go undetected

Down

1. Internet-based program used by hospitals and healthcare systems for documenting, tracking, and trending medication errors

2. error in which any circumstance, action, inaction, or decision related to healthcare contributes to an unintended health result

3. failure resulting from administrative or functional rules, policies, or procedures

5. failure resulting from location or equipment

9. confidential national voluntary program for reporting medication errors

10. error that occurs when two or more options exist and the wrong option is chosen

12. situation that health professionals seek to prevent through root cause analysis

15. error that involves unexpected death or serious physical or psychological injury, or the potential for such occurrences

16. legal standing

Across

2. error whose source or harm includes a drug

4. factor that leads to a medication error if it varies from the correct amount by more than 5%

5. factor that can lead to a medication error if it varies by 30 minutes or more

6. FDA reporting system for adverse events resulting from medications and medical devices

7. factor that leads to a medication error if it varies from the accepted interpretation of the physician's order

8. error in which a prescribed dose is not given

11. institute that has compiled a list of drug names that sound alike or are similar in spelling

12. source or origin of a medication error

13. dose error in which more doses are received by a patient than were prescribed by the physician

14. error that occurs when an essential piece of information cannot be verified and is guessed or presumed

17. error generated by failure that occurs at an individual level

---

Human Relations and Communications

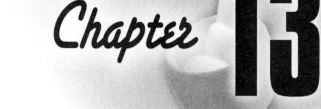

Chapter **13**

COMMUNICATION AND PHARMACY PRACTICE

1. a. Define the following terms as they relate to communication skills:

   1) pronunciation _____

   2) enunciation _____

   3) expression _____

   4) tone _____

   b. Review the terms listed in question 1a. Which ones represent an area of strength for you? On which ones do you need to work?_____

   _____

   _____

2. Pharmacy technicians must be very careful to spell names and medications correctly. Whether you are the speaker or listener, be sure to use verification phrases to check spelling. For example, you might say, "The patient's name begins with *A* as in *Adam*." Make a list of verification phrases that you might use. Be sure to use words or names that will not easily be confused or mistaken for something else.

   A as in _____

   B as in _____

   C as in _____

   D as in _____

   E as in _____

   F as in _____

   G as in _____

   H as in _____

   I as in _____

   J as in _____

Name _____ **Date** _____

K as in _____

L as in _____

M as in _____

N as in _____

O as in _____

P as in _____

Q as in _____

R as in _____

S as in _____

T as in _____

U as in _____

V as in _____

W as in _____

X as in _____

Y as in _____

Z as in _____

3. State what you should do and say in the following situations involving the use of the telephone:

  a. A caller will not terminate the casual conversation that has developed, and you are very busy. _____

     _____

     _____

  b. A caller is angry about the price of his prescription. _____

     _____

     _____

  c. A caller is requesting information about a patient. _____

     _____

     _____

  d. A caller is requesting the pharmacist by her first name, and the pharmacy is very busy. _____

     _____

     _____

  e. You receive a personal phone call from a friend. _____

     _____

     _____

f. You could not understand a caller's speech, and you need him to repeat what he is saying. _____

_____

_____

g. The caller has a medical emergency regarding a prescription drug. _____

_____

_____

h. A caller states that you gave her the wrong medication and she is now very angry. _____

_____

_____

i. A caller is on the phone demanding to speak with the pharmacist NOW.

_____

_____

4. Think of a person you know personally who is a good communicator. List at least five personal characteristics that make him or her an effective communicator. _____

_____

_____

_____

_____

5. What does the phrase "know your personal biases and try to correct them" mean? How will knowing your personal biases help you?_____

_____

_____

_____

6. When a patient has come in person or called to make a complaint regarding the pharmacy, it is important to obtain factual information. Handling complaints and angry patients can be one of the most difficult tasks in the pharmacy. How a complaint is handled will affect whether the patient comes back and whether he or she tells others about the experience.

a. What other types of information, besides factual, will the patient give you that are important? _____

_____

_____

b. How can you show the patient you are taking his or her complaint seriously?_____

_____

_____

c. Why is it important to restate the complaint back to the patient? _____

_____

_____

d. How can you avoid becoming angry with the patient? _____

_____

_____

7. Typically, what do the following behaviors or body postures communicate?

a. finger drumming or tapping one's fingers _____

_____

b. turning away from the speaker as a sentence begins _____

_____

c. repeatedly looking away from the speaker and toward the floor_____

_____

d. repeated sighing_____

_____

e. silence with fingers or hand over the lips _____

_____

8. Make a list of the gestures and body language that you commonly use during a normal day._____

_____

_____

_____

_____

a. What feelings are you communicating with each gesture?

_____

_____

_____

_____

b. Show these gestures to a classmate, and ask him or her to interpret your communication. Do the gestures match what your classmate interpreted?

_____

_____

9. Communication in the pharmacy is very important, both with patients and coworkers. Describe how the following nonverbal cues may help or hinder your communication:

a. eye contact _____

_____

_____

b. body movement such as head nodding and hand gestures _____

_____

_____

c. note taking during the interaction_____

_____

_____

d. clarity of the voice_____

_____

_____

e. tone of the voice _____

_____

_____

f. open-ended questions (e.g., "Explain how…?")_____

_____

_____

g. closed questions (e.g., those inviting a yes-or-no answer) _____

_____

_____

h. repetition of parts of the conversation _____

_____

_____

WEB ACTIVITIES

1. Visit the Exploring Nonverbal Communication Web site, at http://nonverbal.ucsc.edu/, and link to the various previews listed. Test your knowledge and interpretation of the provided samples. List five things you learned about nonverbal communication from other cultures.

2. Type **nonverbal communication** into a search engine of your choice. Many library sites and dictionaries of nonverbal communication are available on-line. Locate a site that has particularly useful information, and write a paragraph describing its contents.

3. Patient confidentiality regulations from the Health Insurance Portability and Accountability Act (HIPAA) of 1996 have had a major effect on all personnel and healthcare facilities. Go to www.hhs.gov/ocr/hipaa and find the following information:

a. the law's major purpose _____

b. the law's key provisions

_____

_____

_____

PUZZLING TERMINOLOGY

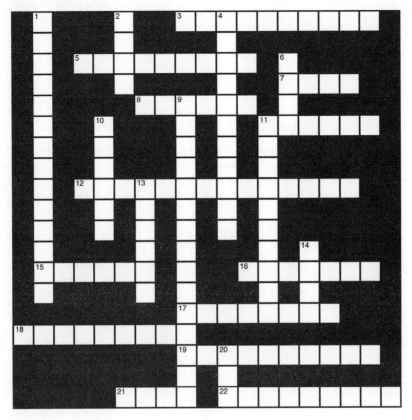

19. patient's name, address, phone number, social security number, or medical identification number

21. language consisting of gestures, movements, and mannerisms

22. unwritten rules of behavior

Down

1. term represented by the first A in HIPAA

2. type of communication that occurs when a technician mumbles or speaks too quickly

4. term represented by the *P* in *HIPAA*

6. characteristic of the voice that is used in nonverbal communication

9. policy of protecting information from unauthorized disclosure

10. set of guidelines for action or behavior in a certain situation

11. mistreatment, sexual or otherwise

13. questions that require a yes-or-no answer

14. type of communication that occurs when a technician speaks clearly and carefully

20. body part that makes contact in visual communication

Across

3. physical look an employee has on the job, including dress and grooming

5. plan for carrying out a particular activity

7. questions that require a descriptive answer, not yes or no

8. unspoken expression involving the mouth, nose, cheeks, and eyes

11. type of information that is protected by HIPAA, including medical diagnoses, medication profiles, and results of laboratory tests

12. preferential treatment or mistreatment

15. ranking of patients for treatment by the priority of their needs

16. behavior that is in good taste

17. disposition a worker adopts toward his or her job duties, customers, employer, and coworkers

18. communication without words

Your Future in Pharmacy Practice

by Jennifer Danielson

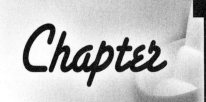

Chapter **14**

COMMUNICATION AND PHARMACY PRACTICE

1. Define *geriatrics*. _____

2. Locate three job postings for a pharmacy technician in your local newspaper or yellow pages, or on the Internet. Identify the position that you would be most interested in pursuing.

3. Adapt the résumé that you prepared in the textbook chapter so that it is appropriate for the specific position you selected in question 1. Write a cover letter to go with the résumé.

4. Describe why each of the following tips is important when interviewing:

   a. Bring an extra copy of your résumé and references to the interview._____

   _____

   b. Bring a written list of three to five questions you wish to ask the interviewer. _____

   _____

   c. Bring a pad of paper and a pen to the interview._____

   _____

   d. Focus on your strengths._____

   _____

   e. Dress professionally for the interview, even if dress is usually casual at this facility. _____

   _____

5. Discuss with a classmate the following ethical dilemmas, and then write a brief statement explaining your opinion on each issue. Write another brief statement outlining a position on the dilemma that is the opposite of your position.

   a. Is there a legitimate need for medical use of marijuana?

   b. How can pharmacy staff participate in pro-choice/pro-life debates?

---

c. What is the pharmacy's obligation to medically uninsured patients?

d. Do patients deserve full disclosure on "near-miss" medication errors?

6. Not much legislation exists regarding technicians providing patient education and training on blood glucose meters. Even though pharmacists are usually the ones to provide specific patient counseling and education, do you think technicians can fulfill this role? Search the Internet to find out whether your state board of pharmacy has a published position on this issue. (Start your search at the National Association of Boards of Pharmacy Web site, www.nabp.net.) Are there any regulations governing such a practice in your area? What is the standard of care for providing such education in your area of practice?

WEB ACTIVITIES

1. Search the Internet for a local workforce development Web site. This site should have information regarding local jobs available.

   a. Where is the local workforce development office located? _____
   _____

   b. What are its hours? _____
   _____

   c. Does your local agency have Internet services? If so, describe them. _____
   _____
   _____
   _____

2. Visit the Pharmacy Technician Certification Board (PTCB) Web site, at www.ptcb.org, and research the recommended texts for PTCE preparation. Locate a short description and pricing information for at least three of the listed texts or references. Prepare a written report to share with your instructor and classmates. Check an interesting article in *CPhT Connection* and share it with the class.

3. Visit the Web site of the hospital or national pharmacy chain with stores nearest to you. Locate where within the site open positions are posted. Locate the mission statement for that organization. If you were to apply for a position with this organization, how would knowing this mission statement help you during the interview?

4. Search the Internet for reputable Web sites reporting news on a pharmacist's right to refuse to fill a prescription because doing so would contradict his or her individual ethical and moral beliefs. What do those participating in the national debate of this issue have to say? Research the position of the national pharmacy associations on this issue. Discuss in a group how you think this affects pharmacy technicians.

PUZZLING TERMINOLOGY

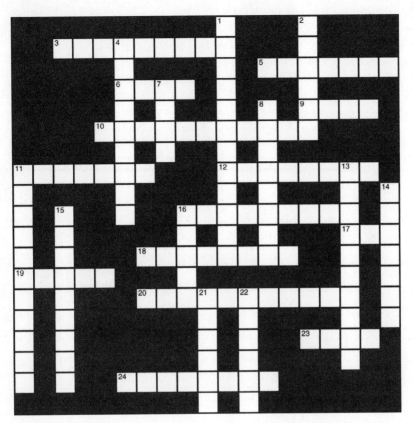

1. process that allows state boards to track technician employment

2. study of standards of conduct and moral judgment that outlines rightness or wrongness of human conduct or character

4. high degree of knowledge in a particular field

7. formal written statement of principles and rules for making decisions about ethical dilemmas

8. principle that motivates someone to think or behave in a moral fashion

11. another word for dependability

13. knowledge and abilities needed to perform a particular job

14. principle of being fair and equitable

15. two-year degree that allows technicians to be given greater responsibilities

16. letter of application

21. conviction that will keep a candidate from sitting for the certification exam for pharmacy technicians

22. brief written summary of what a job candidate has to offer an employer

Across

3. respect due to someone because of his or her superior position

5. dilemma that calls for a judgment between two or more solutions, not all of which are necessarily wrong

6. examination that pharmacy technicians must pass to be certified

9. pharmacy technician who has passed the certification exam

10. documented evidence of qualifications

11. machinery used for repackaging unit doses in many institutional settings

12. freedom from errors

16. what employees should always accept gracefully

17. nonprofit testing company that administers the certification exam for pharmacy technicians

18. formal, binding agreement

19. style of letter in which all items begin at the left margin

20. observable, measurable execution of one's job responsibilities

23. organization that has developed the certification exam for pharmacy technicians

24. state of being self-governing

Drug Identification, Safety, and Information

Appendixes and Resources

COMMUNICATION AND PHARMACY PRACTICE

1. The following real-life medical document contains the technical terms and abbreviations listed on page 195. Define these terms and abbreviations using Appendixes A, B, and C of the textbook, plus a medical dictionary or similar reference.

Camden County Regional Medical Center

32116 Briar Drive Atchley, NC 88976 phone (773) 555-6543 fax (773) 555-4321

Discharge Summary

ADMITTING DIAGNOSIS: New IDDM, juvenile onset

DISCHARGE DIAGNOSIS: New IDDM, juvenile onset

HISTORY OF PRESENT ILLNESS: Patient is a 13 y/o male with a 6-week history of polyuria and polydipsia, nocturia, lethargy, and weight loss. Urine was positive for glucose on admission.

DISCHARGE SUMMARY Page 1	PT. NAME:	TYLER M. MILLER
	ID NO:	IP-851007 - 2415
	ROOM NO:	231
	ADM. DATE:	July 17, 20XX
	DIS. DATE:	July 21, 20XX
	ATT. PHYS:	Keith L. Hamman

(continues)

Name   Date

HOSPITAL COURSE: Patient was admitted to H200 and treated with Regular insulin. Treatment was modified to a 2-shot regimen of NPH and Regular before breakfast and before dinner. By hospital day 3, treatment regimen was established. At that point, there was no hyperglycemia during the day or at night, and symptoms of polyuria, polydipsia, nocturia, and lethargy resolved. Blood sugars stabilized, and there was no overnight hypoglycemia. There were no urine ketones. During the course of hospitalization, the patient, both his parents, and the paternal grandparents underwent instruction in diabetic care, including insulin administration, urine testing, and Accu-Cheks. They were judged to be able to correctly perform all of those activities.

LABORATORY DATA: Laboratory studies at discharge revealed the following: blood glucose: 90, Na: 134, K: 4.1, Cl: 103, CO_2 : 27, BUN 9, creatinine 0.7. Thyroid and liver function tests were unremarkable; glycohemoglobin was 18. Urine was negative for glucose, protein, and ketones.

PHYSICAL EXAMINATION: T: 98.6, P 76, R 17, BP: 110/66. Physical examination was unremarkable and essentially unchanged from admission. Xerosis of hands and perioral area was largely resolved.

DISCHARGE PROGRAM: Pt. will be seen in the clinic in 1 week. He is being discharged on a 2000 cal. ADA diet including three meals and two snacks. He may return to school in 1 week and gradually begin to resume normal activities. He is to check blood glucose at 2 AM for the next two mornings—in addition to regular blood glucose and urine testing—and is to call the clinic each morning for insulin dose adjustments until 7/30/XX.

DISCHARGE MEDICATIONS: Novolin Human Insulin, 10 U. of Regular and 10 U. of NPH 20 min. before breakfast; 10 U. of Regular and 6 U. of NPH 20 minutes before dinner.

———————————————————

Keith L. Hamman, MD

DISCHARGE SUMMARY Page 2	**PT. NAME:** TYLER M. MILLER **ID NO:** IP-851007 - 2415 **ROOM NO:** 231 **ADM. DATE:** July 17, 20XX **DIS. DATE:** July 21, 20XX **ATT. PHYS:** Keith L. Hamman

a. IDDM _____

b. polyuria _____

c. polydipsia _____

d. nocturia _____

e. lethargy _____

f. regular insulin _____

g. NPH insulin _____

h. hypoglycemia _____

i. ketones _____

j. Na _____

k. K _____

l. Cl _____

m. CO_2 _____

n. BUN _____

o. glycohemoglobin _____

p. xerosis _____

q. perioral _____

r. ADA diet _____

s. U _____

t. Novolin _____

2. The following real-life medical document contains the technical terms and abbreviations listed below it. Define these terms and abbreviations using Appendixes A, B, and C of the textbook, plus a medical dictionary or similar reference.

Hayes-Oakwood Clinic, Inc.
Department of Dermatology

407 S. Parkway Accord City, KS 77709-4321
phone (333) 555-1122 fax (333) 555-1234

Physician's Progress Note

PATIENT: Kane, Ronald H.
DATE: February 11, 20XX

<u>S</u>: Patient is a 30 y/o professional accountant. He is unmarried and lives alone. He comes to the clinic today with an extensive rash over his forehead and ears. He reports that the lesions have been present in some degree for the past 4 to 5 months, but have become worse in the past few weeks. He has tried over-the-counter remedies, including various soaps, without relief. Mr. Kane is experiencing a great deal of stress from the breakup of a 6-year relationship with a woman he had expected to marry and believes the stress contributes to his condition.

<u>O</u>: Erythema with greasy, yellow scales, across the entire forehead from hairline to eyebrows. External ears are similarly involved. There are patchy erythematous lesions with scaling along the hairline at the back of the neck. Erythematous papules are scattered across the face, and skin appears quite oily around the nostrils.

<u>A</u>: Seborrheic dermatitis

<u>P</u>: Rx: hydrocortisone cream, 4%, 1 oz tube
Sig: apply to affected areas tid
Patient was counseled on avoiding stress and stress-relieving measures, because that aggravates his condition. He was instructed to avoid soap on the area and to use only an oatmeal cleansing bar on his face. He is to also avoid over-the-counter preparations. He is to RTC in 4 weeks if the condition is not greatly improved.

---

a. SOAP _____

b. lesions _____

c. erythema _____

d. papules _____

e. seborrheic dermatitis_____

f. tid _____

g. RTC_____

3. The following real-life medical document contains the technical terms and abbreviations listed on page 198. Define these terms and abbreviations using Appendixes A, B, and C of the textbook, plus a medical dictionary or similar reference.

Clinic Note

PATIENT: Daniel Caine
DATE: July 13, 20XX

S: 36 y/o white male reports increasing night sweats, low back pain, headaches, persistent cough, lack of appetite, and general malaise. Denies polyuria, hematuria, and states he believes his long-standing cystitis may be better this week. He states that he easily becomes fatigued and often has difficulty sleeping. Patient states, "It is so hard to get up in the morning, most days I just stay in bed." He is unemployed and living with his parents following his diagnosis of HIV infection in 1999. He continues to be followed by Dr. Henry Timmons in Chicago for treatment of his primary diagnosis and receives AZT; he reports taking that medication as directed. Patient states that in the past 3 months his CD4 count, which has been decreasing, seems to have stabilized. The count is still low, however, with an absolute value of 260. He acknowledges additional diagnoses of chronic active hepatitis, chronic cystitis, oral candidiasis, and depression. His depression is currently being treated with Triavil, and he reports taking that medication as directed. He states that he has stopped smoking, as of last month, and does not consume ETOH. He is seen in the clinic today for routine follow-up.

O: Patient is thin, pale, and appears somewhat fragile. Movements and speech are somewhat slow. Vital signs: T 98 F, P 88, R 24, BP 142/88. Supraclavicular lymph nodes are enlarged and shotty. Oral mucosa is slightly reddened but appears otherwise normal. There is no leukoplakia. Mild bilateral wheezing on expiration. Left side of abdomen is soft and nontender; right side is mildly tender. No suprapubic tenderness. Liver margin is palpable approximately 2 cm below the costal margin; hepatomegaly is unchanged since last exam. Back is slightly tender to palpation throughout the lumbar area. Remainder of examination is unremarkable.

A: 1) HIV infection
   2) Chronic hepatitis B
   3) Chronic depression; not responding well to current therapy
   4) Chronic cystitis
   5) Chronic oral candidiasis infection

P: 1) Patient will continue AZT therapy and will continue to be followed by Dr. Timmons
   2) Zoloft, 50 mg, 1 qAM
   3) Routine clinic labs
   4) Social worker to discuss appropriate short- and long-term goals with patient and explore aspects of depression

_____

Leroy F. Cincaid, MD

---

a. y/o _____

b. malaise _____

c. polyuria _____

d. hematuria _____

e. cystitis _____

f. HIV _____

g. AZT _____

h. CD4 _____

i. hepatitis _____

j. candidiasis _____

k. ETOH _____

l. supraclavicular _____

m. oral mucosa _____

n. leukoplakia _____

o. bilateral wheezing _____

p. expiration _____

q. suprapubic _____

r. palpable _____

s. costal _____

t. lumbar _____

4. Use Appendix B to define the following prefixes:

a. a- _____

b. bi- _____

c. brady- _____

d. dys- _____

e. extra- _____

f. hyper- _____

g. intra- _____

h. peri- _____

i. post- _____

j. re- _____

k. sub- _____

l. trans- _____

m. anti- _____

n. epi- _____

o. dia- _____

p. ex-_____

q. hemi- _____

r. inter- _____

s. mal- _____

t. poly-_____

u. pre-_____

v. retro- _____

w. tachy-_____

x. uni-_____

5. Use Appendix B to define the following root word parts:

a. aden/o _____

b. ur/o _____

c. rhin/o_____

d. enter/o_____

e. ren/o _____

f. hem/o _____

g. viscer/o _____

h. cardi/o_____

i. cyst/o_____

j. oste/o_____

6. Use Appendix B to define the following suffixes:

a. -algia _____

b. -ism _____

c. -osis _____

d. -sclerosis _____

e. -uria _____

f. -emia _____

g. -itis_____

h. -rhea_____

i. -pathy_____

j. -centesis_____

Go to the student Internet Resource Center (IRC) for *Pharmacy Practice for Technicians, Third Edition,* at www.emcp.com, and click on the Resources link in the Readings in Subject Area sidebar. This provides a listing of pharmacy resources with hotlinks to their associated Web sites. Use those resources to respond to the following questions and activities.

7. Write out the following abbreviations and briefly describe each organization:

a. AAPT _____

_____

b. APhA _____

_____

c. ASHP _____

_____

d. DEA _____

_____

e. FDA _____

_____

f. NABP _____

_____

g. NACDS _____

_____

h. NCPA _____

_____

i. PTCB _____

_____

j. USP _____

_____

8. Provide an example of each of the following items. Get the information from a package insert for a widely used prescription medication, or look up this information in a current edition of *Physician's Desk Reference (PDR)*.

a. brand name _____

b. generic name _____

c. manufacturer _____

d. indications _____

e. method of administration _____

f. dose forms available _____

g. contraindications _____

h. potential for abuse or dependence _____

9. Using *Remington: The Science and Practice of Pharmacology,* look up and then describe how to compound a standard rectal suppository. _____

_____

_____

10. Look up the drug chlorambucil in the *United States Pharmacopeia* or a reference of your choice. Then answer the following questions:

a. What type of drug is chlorambucil, and what is its primary indication?

_____

_____

b. What precautions should be taken when handling this drug? _____

_____

_____

_____

c. How should the drug be packaged and stored? _____

_____

_____

d. What reference can be used to identify the shape, color, and other characteristics of chlorambucil tablets? _____

_____

11. Using reference works listed on the Resources link for this course at the student Internet Resource Center (IRC), find a recent journal article on the subject of recertification of pharmacy technicians.

a. What is the title of the article? _____

_____

b. Identify the authors. _____

_____

c. Read the article, then, on your own paper, write a few paragraphs explaining the point of view of the article. Give three reasons for your agreement or disagreement with it.

12. Where can you find the signs, symptoms, and treatments for appendicitis? What are they? _____

_____

_____

_____

13. Are Lasix (furosemide) and potassium chloride (KCl) compatible in the same IV bag? Why or why not? What source did you use to answer this question?

_____

_____

14. Do Percocet and Roxicet contain the same ingredients or different ingredients? What are the ingredients? What source did you use to answer these questions?

_____

_____

15. What is the address of the Parke-Davis Company? What source did you use to answer this question? _____

    _____

    _____

16. A prescription for green soap has come into the pharmacy. Where will you find the instructions for making it? What are those ingredients? _____

    _____

    _____

17. How many milligrams and milliequivalents of calcium are in 1 g of calcium gluceptate? What source did you use to answer the question? _____

    _____

    _____

18. What reference book contains information on the evolution of pharmacy, ethics of pharmacy, chemical applications of pharmacy applications, and pharmacy law? _____

    _____

19. In what strengths is Zaroxolyn available? What source did you use to answer the question? _____

    _____

    _____

20. What is the pediatric dose of chloramphenicol? How will it be dispensed? What source did you use to answer these questions? _____

    _____

    _____

21. What reference would best describe how a local anesthetic works? _____

    _____

22. What is another brand name for Motrin? What source did you use to answer the question? _____

    _____

23. What is another name for Hyserp? For what is it indicated? What source did you use to answer the question? _____

    _____

    _____

24. What is the phone number for AstraZeneca Pharmaceuticals, Inc.? What source did you use to answer this question? _____

    _____

25. What reference would show the chemical structure of paraldehyde and give information regarding packaging and storage? What are the storage instructions?

_____

_____

26. What reference would explain the "controlled substance" labeling? _____

_____

27. Your instructor will present five drug products; locate the resource that will assist you in identifying the products._____

_____

28. Review pharmacy journals published in the last 6 months, and answer the following questions regarding five different drug advertisements:

   a. What is the drug name? _____

     _____

   b. What is the source (periodical name, issue, and page number)? _____

     _____

   c. What caught your eye in this advertisement?_____

     _____

   d. Was the advertisement educational in any way? What did you learn?_____

     _____

29. Use the reference *Drug Facts and Comparisons* to answer the following questions:

   a. What is the brand name for azithromycin?_____

     _____

   b. What is Relafen indicated for?_____

     _____

   c. What strengths does Dilantin (caps and tabs) come in?_____

     _____

   d. Is Zoloft indicated for post-traumatic stress disorder?_____

     _____

   e. What is Zestril indicated for?_____

     _____

   f. What warnings should accompany tetracycline? _____

     _____

   g. Premarin has what major contraindications? _____

     _____

   h. Boniva should be taken in what manner? How often? _____

     _____

i. What is the brand name of a rabies vaccination? _____

_____

j. Namenda is used for patients with what disease? _____

_____

WEB ACTIVITIES

1. Visit MedicineNet.com, at www.medicinenet.com/Script/Main/hp.asp, and look for the site's medical terminology dictionary.

   a. Is the dictionary user friendly? Why or why not? _____

   _____

   _____

   b. Would you recommend that patients use this site to learn about medical terms? Why or why not?_____

   _____

   _____

2. Check your recall of drug names by using the flash cards or crossword puzzles provided in the Study Hall section for this course at the student Internet Resource Center (IRC), www.emcp.com.

   a. If you choose Top Rx Drugs Interactive Flash Cards, you will see flash cards with the generic names of the most commonly prescribed drugs, and you will have an opportunity to guess their brand names.

   b. If you choose Games, you will be given crossword puzzles with clues consisting of generic names or brand names, and asked to supply the corresponding brand names or generic names. See how many drugs you can correctly identify.

3. On the Resources link for this course at the student Internet Resource Center (IRC), create bookmarks or favorites on your browser to link to the resources that you think will be most helpful. Write a summary of why you selected these sites.

4. Visit www.healthweb.org/ and click on three different areas of interest to you. Prepare a summary report on each area. How do you see using this site in your personal life?

5. Visit www.medweb.emory.edu/MedWeb/ and click on several options in the Consumer Health area. Report on what is currently available in terms of information for the general public.

6. Visit Healthtouch Online, at www.healthtouch.com/.

   a. What is the definition of Healthtouch Online? _____

   _____

   _____

b. What can be found in the Medication Guide?_____

_____

_____

c. What is the Health Resource Directory?_____

_____

_____

d. What happens if you click on one of the organizations listed in the Health Resource Directory? _____

_____

_____

7. Visit www.hon.ch/, the Health on the Net (HON) site. The Health on the Net Foundation, created in 1995, is a not-for-profit international organization operating out of Geneva, Switzerland. HON's mission is to guide laypeople or nonmedical users and medical practitioners to useful and reliable on-line medical and health information. HON provides leadership in setting ethical standards for Web site developers.

a. What is the advantage of using sites that have the HON logo on them?

_____

_____

b. What types of media are in the multimedia center? _____

_____

_____

c. In how many languages can you search medical words? _____

_____

_____

PUZZLING TERMINOLOGY

Preventing Prescription Errors

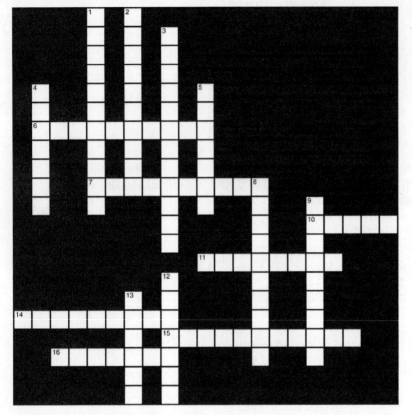

Down

1. form of a new drug name that should be previewed by pharmacists to determine whether it is easily confused with another drug name

2. characteristic of a drug name that can be changed through manipulation of boldface, color, and/or capital letters

3. method for emphasizing text on a computer screen or printout

4. "name alert" indicator that can be affixed in an area where look-alike or sound-alike products are stored

5. process of keeping track of medication errors

8. tool that puts a drug order or prescription at eye level, where it may be easier to read

9. tool that can help you read small print on a drug order or prescription

12. person who should see an easily confused medication and hear cautions about it before accepting it

13. process of communicating information about medication errors

Across

6. product information that should be supplied on all outpatient prescriptions and inpatient drug orders

7. form of a prescription that can prevent confusion with drug names

10. signal indicating that one of a pair of easily confused drug names has been entered into the computer

11. environmental feature that can be regulated to enhance the readability of drug orders and prescriptions

14. areas where look-alike or sound-alike products should be stored

15. check in which one person interprets and enters the prescription into the computer, and another reviews the printed label against the original prescription and the product

16. characteristic that can help you determine which of two look-alike or sound-alike drugs to dispense or administer

Look-Alike, Sound-Alike Drug Names

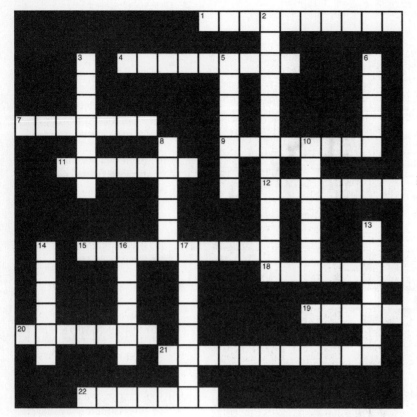

19. drug name easily confused with Lasix

20. drug name easily confused with Xeloda

21. drug name easily confused with aripiprazole

22. drug name easily confused with Serophene

Down

2. drug name easily confused with morphine

3. drug name easily confused with Toradol

5. drug name easily confused with Ultracet

6. drug name easily confused with Paxil

8. drug name easily confused with Allegra

10. drug name easily confused with Atacand

13. drug name easily confused with Precare

14. drug name easily confused with Zantac

16. drug name easily confused with Norcuron

17. drug name easily confused with methadone

Across

1. drug name easily confused with Brethine

4. drug name easily confused with Dilaudid

7. drug name easily confused with ketorolac

9. drug name easily confused with Colazal

11. drug name easily confused with ritodrine

12. drug name easily confused with Platinol

15. drug name easily confused with gentian violet

18. drug name easily confused with Indocid